2/01/06

Bow 9/06
MIN 8/07
Cta 11/08
Svatt 10/10 8/13
Sbott 12/116
CW 419

S0-AID-960

CAESAR'S HOURS

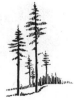

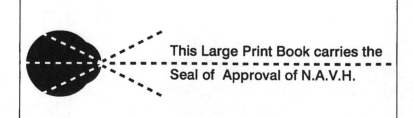

CAESAR'S HOURS

My Life in Comedy,
with Love and Laughter

SID CAESAR
WITH EDDY FRIEDFELD

Thorndike Press • Waterville, Maine

Published in 2004 by arrangement with
Public Affairs, a member of Perseus Books LLC.

Thorndike Press® Large Print Biography.

The tree indicium is a trademark of Thorndike Press.

The text of this Large Print edition is unabridged.
Other aspects of the book may vary from the original edition.

Set in 16 pt. Plantin.

Printed in the United States on permanent paper.

Library of Congress Cataloging-in-Publication Data

Caesar, Sid, 1922–
    Caesar's hours : my life in comedy, with love and
    laughter / Sid Caesar with Eddy Friedfeld.
      p. cm.
    Originally published: New York : Public Affairs, 2003.
    ISBN 0-7862-6345-8 (lg. print : hc : alk. paper)
    1. Caesar, Sid, 1922– 2. Entertainers — United States
  — Biography. I. Friedfeld, Eddy. II. Title.
PN2287.C22A3 2004
791.4502′8′092—dc22
  [B]   2003071192

To my late brother David, who had confidence in my artistic ability before anyone else did, and who always encouraged me.
Dave, I miss you every day.

To my wife, Florence, who taught me how to live, how to breathe, and how to dream.

And to my writers, for all the love and laughter.

SID CAESAR

To my late grandmother, Rosa Friedfeld, who first introduced me to the magic of Sid Caesar. Thank you for that and for everything else.

EDDY FRIEDFELD

As the Founder/CEO of NAVH, the only national health agency solely devoted to those who, although not totally blind, have an eye disease which could lead to serious visual impairment, I am pleased to recognize Thorndike Press★ as one of the leading publishers in the large print field.

Founded in 1954 in San Francisco to prepare large print textbooks for partially seeing children, NAVH became the pioneer and standard setting agency in the preparation of large type.

Today, those publishers who meet our standards carry the prestigious "Seal of Approval" indicating high quality large print. We are delighted that Thorndike Press is one of the publishers whose titles meet these standards. We are also pleased to recognize the significant contribution Thorndike Press is making in this important and growing field.

Lorraine H. Marchi, L.H.D.
Founder/CEO
NAVH

★ Thorndike Press encompasses the following imprints: Thorndike, Wheeler, Walker and Large Pr int Press.

CONTENTS

Part Three
A LEGACY IN COMEDY

INTRODUCTION

Thanks to his phenomenal physical stamina, which was always at the service of his miraculous mental machinery, the wonder is that the small screen ever could contain Sid Caesar at all.

Some men are born with the ability to pitch a strikeout to any man at the plate. Some are born with the ability to outbox, outrun, and outthink all other men. Sid Caesar was born with the ability to be all other men. He had only to don a costume, add a mole, a mustache, or a monocle, then assume the right accent and attitudes, and he was able to portray, with dead-on accuracy, anyone from a suburbanite to a Samurai, from a king to a cobbler, from a duke to a drunk. Anyone that we, his writers (and total fans), would ask Sid to be, he would obligingly, killingly funny, be.

Sadly, the only man Sid ever had trouble being — the one character that eluded him

9

for years — was Sid himself. Troubled as he was for far too much of his life, Sid just didn't seem to be able to work his way to the front of the line of all of the countless characters he'd created to hide behind.

He could break your heart in the role of a silent movie star whose career went south with the advent of sound. He could re-break it, as he did in a mock opera in which he sang and played (all in largely improvised Italian double-talk) the part of "Galipacci," a clown forced to hide his tears from the circus audience.

That particular role best typified Sid's own inability to articulate, or in any way reveal, the inner man, the real Sid Caesar. So difficult was the task, that whenever he was required to speak in his own voice to express his own feelings, he often made ordinary English sound like so much improvised double-talk. Obliged to greet the audience at the start of each show — it was *Caesar's Hour* after all — Sid would struggle desperately with a simple, "Good evening, ladies and gentlemen." There were nights when those few short words threatened to turn into a miniseries of their own.

If any of this sounds harsh or critical, be assured that however crazy Sid was, we, his writers, were even crazier about him. There were no "don'ts" in the Writers' Room. Except for maybe don't be boring and, for sure, don't ever stop trying to come up with stuff that only Sid could do. When you've got a Mozart on your hands, you don't write "Chopsticks" for him to perform. Show in and show out, we were encouraged to come up with the freshest, most challenging material we could think of. Sid was performing takeoffs on Japanese films long before he ever saw one.

His gift to those of us who gathered in that room was to offer us the challenge of discovering who *we* were — or who we might possibly become — as writers.

LARRY GELBART

MY FIRST LAUGH

The first laugh I ever got on a stage was when I was eleven years old in the assembly hall at Nathaniel Hawthorne Junior High School in Yonkers, New York. I had never even been in front of an audience before. I was playing saxophone in the school band at the time. The music teacher liked my tone and my phrasing, so she picked me to play a solo of "The Swan" by Camille Saint-Saëns.

You can imagine what a big deal it was to be chosen to play a solo in front of the entire school at a musical night to which families were invited. I rehearsed with a young girl who accompanied me on the piano, and I was plenty nervous.

That night, parents, relatives, and friends filled the school auditorium, including my parents and my two brothers, Abe and Dave. I was still wearing knickers. I nervously walked out onto the stage and stood in front of the folding music stand

12

with my music next to the piano. I looked over and gave the young girl the nod to start playing the piano.

All of a sudden, just as I was about to start playing, something blinded me. It was the spotlight, directly on me. I had never been in the spotlight before; all I knew was the light was so bright, I couldn't see the music. So I walked five or six steps to my right, carrying the music stand over a few feet.

I was about to start playing and bang! The spotlight hit me in the eyes again. I carried the music stand back to where I was originally, but the spotlight followed in the same blinding way and I still couldn't see the music. I waved to the spotlight guy and walked the other way, again carrying the stand. People in the audience started to snicker.

I heard the snickering and the commotion and thought, "Hey, this might be funny." So I started playing tag with the spotlight. More people in the audience started to laugh. I faked a move to the left, then to the right, playing the moment. The snickering grew into out-and-out laughter. The spotlight guy finally got the message and turned the light off.

I played my solo and got a nice round of

applause. After the show, I met my parents outside the auditorium. My father asked me, "Why were you making such a fool of yourself, running back and forth? People were laughing at you. Why would you do that?"

"Pop, you don't understand," I told him. "The spotlight was in my eyes. I couldn't see the music."

I looked at my brother Dave. "You were pretty good," he told me. He could not have been prouder of me. My mother and both my brothers knew that the audience was laughing with me, not at me. My father also figured it out a short while later. It was that night that I discovered that I could make strangers laugh in public.

The best thing about humor is that it shows people they're not alone. Once I did a sketch about an accident-prone man getting up in the morning. There really are accident-prone people in the world. Just seeing that there are others out there like you is a comfort. I played a man who woke up in the morning and stretched. I hear and feel a pop. Pow! A shoulder goes out of whack. First thing in the morning! Everybody's human and everyone wants to be like other humans. They want that connection.

My yardstick, my litmus test for anything I did creatively, was that it had to have a basis in reality. It had to be believable. All my comedy was character and plot driven. I always believed that in art and life, it's not what you do, it's the way you do it; it's not what you say, it's the way you say it. In the doing you'll find your strengths and weaknesses, and you will find your art.

I always wanted to be Charlie Chaplin. He was one of my earliest comedic heroes, along with Buster Keaton, Laurel and Hardy, and W. C. Fields. Most of their comedy came from their character. They each believed in what they did, and I believed them.

The essence of their humor was what I call "working both sides of the street" — a mixture of comedy and pathos. They blended comedy and drama in such a way that you laughed, but you also felt something passionate in your heart. Everything in life is a combination of something else. There's no "one thing" that forms your personality. When you're growing up, you develop as an individual by unconsciously assimilating a little bit from your parents, your siblings, relatives, and friends. The same process holds true for the development of the creative personality.

Charlie Chaplin was a great pantomimist,

a great acrobat, and he knew the value of combining comedy and pathos. For example, how would you make a blind girl in a silent movie think you're very rich in a split second? In *City Lights*, Chaplin's little tramp character is always being chased by cops. In one scene, he sees a group of cars backed up for a red light. In a move that has been used many times since, Chaplin runs through the backseats of the cars, out of one car door and into another, crossing the street to elude the law.

The last car he gets out of is a limousine, and on the sidewalk nearby is a blind girl selling violets, who turns toward the sound of the slamming limousine door, thinking that a very rich man must be getting out. Chaplin sees her and instantly falls in love. He takes out his last dime and gives it to the blind girl to buy the violets.

When she goes over to the water fountain to rinse out her cup, Chaplin follows her with love in his eyes. She rinses the cup and then throws the water in his face.

There was a hush in the audience because they didn't know whether to laugh or to cry. That to me was a great piece of comedy because Chaplin captured that bittersweet moment, and was truly working both sides of the street.

Buster Keaton taught me a different lesson. The classic scene where an entire house falls on top of him took not only genius to conceive but also a lot of guts to execute. He had to stand in the exact spot where the attic window would come down over him, so he would not be injured when the whole side of the house fell. The slightest wind deviation could have killed him. That's what I call believing in yourself. Keaton taught me the value of preparation for life and for anything you do because not only did the joke depend on it, so did his life.

Years later, I got to work with Keaton in *It's a Mad, Mad, Mad, Mad World.* We did a scene together in which he was supposed to direct a car backing out of a garage. He had no dialogue. On the spot, Keaton created an unscripted ballet that came directly from his head. He danced around and found pieces of business and turned a simple move of backing the car out into a beautifully funny piece. I watched him create right in front of my eyes and stood there in awe.

I modeled my sketch comedy after Laurel and Hardy. I will never forget how they pushed a piano up dozens of flights of stairs in *The Music Box*. They would set up those kinds of situations, and they would find so many variations of whatever they were doing. Those scenarios were very well thought out and rehearsed and they were able to shoot them in one or two days.

Laurel and Hardy were also extremely sympathetic characters. In one piece set right after World War I, Laurel is in a veterans hospital, sitting on a bench with his leg tucked under him. Hardy comes in to visit and thinks his friend has lost his leg in the war. Hardy is very emotional, saying, "How are you? How are you feeling?" Laurel obliviously responds, "I'm all right."

Hardy thinks that his friend is putting up a brave front. "Why don't we have some lunch?" "Oh that's a good idea." Before Laurel can move, Hardy picks him up and carries him to the restaurant with loving arms. And Laurel just looks up and smiles.

Hardy puts his friend down in the chair in the restaurant. They order and eat. After Hardy pays the bill, Laurel says, "I've got to go to the bathroom." Hardy is about to get up to carry him, but Laurel just gets up and walks by himself.

Hardy does his slow burn and then starts chasing Laurel, yelling at him, "Why did you let me carry you!" In addition to the laughs, the sketch was believable and contained a lot of genuine emotion. At certain points you felt sorry for Hardy because he truly thought his best friend had lost a leg in the war. It showed the kind of care and deep friendship he felt for Laurel.

W. C. Fields' work taught me the essence of comic timing. He was constantly muttering, which was his main comedic prop. There is a classic scene where he is seated in an airplane next to a window. He takes a bottle from which he just sipped and rests it on the windowsill. When the bottle falls out of the window, without any hesitation, he follows the bottle right out of the window. As he is going out the window, he mutters, "Why did I put it on the window?" It was one of the funniest scenes I have ever seen. I learned how to make a scene larger or smaller, how to grow and develop a laugh through using my body and contorting and manipulating my facial expressions.

Fortunately I was able to pick from the best. As Sir Isaac Newton said of his own achievements, "If I have seen further it is by standing on the shoulders of Giants." I, too, stand on the shoulders of giants. It was by learning from these people that I was able to craft my own style.

Nobody does anything alone. There's always someone who showed or gave them something. It's all about what you want to absorb. Your style comes from those to whom you are exposed and from whom you learn. You take all your influences, mix them into a creative milkshake, and assimilate them into your own personality.

I learned to think of life as a camera: It's what you choose to photograph that becomes part of your emotional album. Something can be enlightening or it can be dark and depressing. It's only after you make friends with yourself that you learn these things. Only you know how to press those buttons and turn your emotions on and off.

It's analogous to a general who studies great battles. He would never go into war and use the same battle scenario twice. The other side would recognize the pattern, and it would be a recipe for defeat. It's also the same way in music. Phrasing is a function of a variation on the theme, which creates a style.

When a comedian steps out onto a stage, he never knows whether he is going to do well. Making people laugh is the lifeblood of a comedian. That's why success onstage is taken to extremes. To a professional who is passionate about his craft, each performance takes on life-and-death significance, so much so that it becomes the language of the comedian. When we do well, we "killed the audience," and if we don't succeed and don't connect with the audience, we "died" onstage.

Freud said that humor is a way of dealing with our fears. I always believed that great comedy derives from tragedy and from humanity. There's a fine line between laughter and tears. When you laugh too hard, you start to cry. When you cry too hard, you start to laugh. When someone doesn't know whether to laugh or cry, your comedy is working. Even before Freud, there was an Englishman named William Shakespeare. He was way ahead of his time. He identified everything as a symbol.

I wasn't born funny. I didn't come out of the womb and say, "Good evening Mom and Dad. A funny thing happened on the way to my birth." It's all about hard work and development. Too many people have great talent but lack the drive or discipline to develop it.

I was, and to a certain degree still am, a painfully shy person. Offstage, I was never the life of the party. But in front of a camera, immersing myself in a character, I was able to come alive. Live television was like the opening night of a Broadway show every week. Only on Broadway, there are only fifteen hundred people and a few critics and the material has been tested and honed on the road for months. With us, the material hadn't yet been written five days before — and 60 million people were watching.

You learn nothing from success; you only learn from failure. You will be taken to task many times and you will have to learn from understanding what you did wrong and why. If you do catch yourself doing something right, grab it and try to understand and learn. If you are truly serious about your art, you will study your mistakes, but you won't be discouraged by them.

On television, you are in front of millions of people and thousands of critics. Imagine yourself standing alone in front of 60 million people live; you realize that you have to do something. You're a solo. There's nobody up there but you. You've got to make 60 million people laugh. If you let it get to you, it will scare the hell out of you. But you go with it. Every time you walk out onstage, you tell yourself, now I am going to do my best. All I can see is the audience in front of me. You steel yourself so you can stand up there and do it. That's how I taught myself.

Over fifty years ago, I worked with some of the greatest writers and performers in the history of entertainment. We were young and hard-working and had been thrust into a creative pressure cooker that sounds impossible by today's standards: Write, memorize, craft, and execute ninety minutes of live television each week, not for twenty or twenty-two weeks, but for thirty-nine weeks a year. We didn't know it could not be done, so we did it.

Part 1
PORTRAIT OF THE COMEDIAN AS A YOUNG MAN

Chapter 1

A YONKERS CHILDHOOD

My wife, Florence, always says that a comedian is usually an only child or the youngest child, because both are intent on getting the attention of their parents. It was certainly true in my case.

I was born in Yonkers, then a rough factory town on the Hudson River just north of New York City, on September 8, 1922. I am told it was a bleak day. Me, I don't remember. My parents, Max and Ida, thought of naming me Felix, after Felix Frankfurter, the famous Harvard law professor who later became the first Jewish United States Supreme Court justice. My mother was a little worried about the similarity to Felix the Cat and my being made fun of. So Sidney it was.

I was the youngest of three brothers. Abe was eighteen years older, Dave was ten years older. Not only that, Dave was six feet two inches tall and Abe was a towering six feet four. I was born into a family of giants. Between Abe and Dave, I had another brother, Milton, who died of meningitis at the age of twelve, before I was born.

I believe that I was a "makeup child," which meant my parents had a fight and were mad at each other for a while. During the passion of reconciliation, I was conceived. My father was nearly fifty when I was born and was much older than my mother. My parents never talked about how and where they met. They grew up at a time where romance wasn't necessarily part of marriage. That's a marked contrast to my own marriage, which was and still is all about romance.

My father, Max, came to this country from Poland when he was nine years old, in the late 1880s. Caesar, the name given to him by the immigration officer at Ellis Island, was typical of the jokes that the immigration officers would play on Eastern European immigrants. The family name could have originally been Kaiser or Saiserovich. No one ever remembered for sure.

Max grew up on Broome Street on the Lower East Side of Manhattan, back when they still had sailboats arriving in New York harbor. Although he was only five feet seven and heavyset, Max exuded authority and was a tough, powerful, and stern man. Max was a product of the American immigrant ethic of working hard to get ahead. He was also part of a generation of stoic men who didn't express their feelings openly.

My father was ambitious and industrious. During his youth he held down many eclectic jobs, including being a "Shabbos Goy," which literally meant "Sabbath Gentile." For a penny, he would turn on lights and stoves for more observant Jews who did not perform such activities on the Sabbath.

He later came up with another lucrative endeavor. For fifty cents a day, he would take your new pair of shoes and walk around in them for you, breaking them in. His big feet would stretch the tough leather, and in two days the shoes were comfortable.

My father eventually gave up leather and lights for the food business. He and his older brother Joe opened a luncheonette in Manhattan that they would own and operate for a number of years. He later looked for a place in the up-and-coming town of Yonkers and opened the St. Claire Buffet and Luncheonette on the corner of Riverdale and Main Streets. It catered to workers from the Otis Elevator Company (which alone took up over fifteen square blocks of space), the phone company, the sugar company, and the local carpet and hat factories. There were a lot of mouths that needed to be fed.

The restaurant also had seventy-five rooms for rent upstairs. Rooms without windows cost fifty cents a night. Rooms with windows and a fire escape cost seventy-five cents. The fire escape was a rope tied to the radiator.

My mother, Ida, was a tall and beautiful woman who came to the United States from Russia when she was a year old. She doted on me. I remember her strong body and her dark bobbed hair. She would sing to me in Yiddish and feed me oatmeal.

The restaurant was a twenty-four-hour-a-day operation, and it took my entire family to run it. Abe worked as the counterman from 6:00 a.m. to 6:00 p.m. Dave took over for him from 6:00 p.m. to 6:00 a.m. My mother worked as cashier during lunch. When my mother was gone, Dave was in charge of watching me.

To undercut the competition, my father would get up at three o'clock every morning and drive all the way to the produce market in downtown Manhattan in order to get there before it opened at four.

By 5:45 he was back in Yonkers with a truckload of vegetables in time to serve breakfast to the factory workers. He would often fortify himself against the early morning cold by drinking a tumbler of whiskey laced with spoons of black pepper. Let Starbucks try and match that.

My maternal grandfather, Sam Rafael, was six feet four, which is undoubtedly where the tall genes in the family came from. When he came to the United States, he became a jeweler and repaired watches. He was a bandmaster in the old country, which also accounted for the musical genes. My maternal grandmother, Rachel, spoke very little English but could always make herself understood.

As a young child I would go to Asbury Park, New Jersey, at least two or three times a year, including every summer, to visit my grandparents. Asbury Park was next to Ocean Grove and had a boardwalk, a salt-water swimming pool, and a convention hall, with Skee-Ball and other arcade games. Above the stove in my grandmother's kitchen I remember she had a picture she loved and adored. It was a picture of a Swift's Ham. She was kosher, but she thought it was a very beautiful picture and put it up.

Ocean Grove was a very upscale, happy, and very religious Christian town. But the people couldn't have been that happy, because when they drained the fountain and pond at Ocean Grove there were literally thousands of empty liquor bottles, where the supposedly temperate community used to dump what they weren't supposed to be drinking.

The summer I was six years old I was sent to Asbury Park to meet my mother, who had left a week earlier to be with my grandparents. She liked to stay at a rooming house called Linky's. Dave took me down to Pennsylvania Station in Manhattan and put me on the train to New Jersey. He put a big sign around my neck that said Asbury Park/Ocean Grove. The conductor couldn't miss me. There couldn't have been more fanfare if I was being sent to Europe.

I remember it was raining hard as the train pulled into Asbury Park. I also remember seeing my mother getting onto another train in the other direction, heading back to Manhattan. In those days telephones were only used in an emergency and there was obviously some confusion as to when I was coming. Linky, already at the train station after dropping my mother off, took me back to his rooming house. He put me up and taught me how to play rummy for a couple of days until arrangements were made to get me back to Yonkers.

When I was getting off the train at Penn Station on my way home, a porter grabbed my bags and carried them. "Gee, how nice is this guy," I thought, not yet familiar with the art of tipping. Dave was there to meet me and handed the porter a dime. "You're a big sport with my money," he laughed.

My family was very laughter oriented. Everyone loved to entertain. I remember my father taking me to the Loews Proctors, a Yonkers theater, to watch a vaudeville show. A three-man trio had just finished a song. As they went off the stage to applause, my father turned to me and said, "That must be a very hard song. It takes three people to sing it."

When I was three years old and company would come over, I would sit at the rolltop desk in the living room, take a pencil and paper, and pretend to write diligently. The relatives were duly impressed. They would say, "He's three years old and can read and write." "Not exactly," my father would reply, smiling.

My extended family was funny, too. My mother's sister Alice lived in Harlem with her husband, who was both a dentist and a lawyer. Many a time he had to sue himself. Whenever we would visit them, Alice would put out a one-ounce bag of Planters peanuts and a half a bottle of Pepsi and tell the entire family, "Help yourselves, dig in. Eat what you want." Her husband gave me a World War I helmet, which I cherished for years. My father had a copy of a 1914 edition of *Collier's* magazine that had pictures of military equipment, including machine guns, artillery, and the helmet.

My mother's brother, Ray Rafael, was also a great source of humor. Uncle Ray was a successful businessman who owned a tie factory. He had a strong personality and a wonderful sense of style. He shopped at Phil Kronfeld's, a well-known high-end men's clothing store in Manhattan off of Duffy Square. His shirts were white on white with a roll collar. His initials were monogrammed not only on his shirt and handkerchiefs but also on his socks. When he went to Florida, he took a special train. He would always come visit us in Yonkers in a big late-model car. I heard Ray use the line: "I made it back from Miami in nineteen hours and only hit one red light" long before comedian Gene Bayloos made it famous.

When Ray came to town, everything was open. The family would go out and no matter what we did, there was a lot of laughter because Ray was a great story-teller. He was like the character from Alaska in *Death of a Salesman*, who was marveled at for how he had succeeded.

But the most important person in my life during my childhood was my brother Dave. The joy, the warmth, and the humor of those days came mostly from him. Dave was the funniest, the most good-hearted, and the finest man I ever knew. He was much funnier than I was, but in front of an audience he froze. Dave was not only a genuinely funny person; he was also a gen-uine person. Other than my wife, Florence, no one took more interest in me or took better care of me in my life than Dave.

Dave started me on my way, encouraged me, nurtured and supported me, not only as a brother but also as a best friend, creative muse, and mentor. He was my surrogate father and my one-man cheering section. Having said that, I still believe I am not giving Dave enough credit. Without him, I would not have had the encouragement and support I needed to be an entertainer and an artist. I owe my creative life to my brother Dave, may he rest in peace. Dave had a warm and endearing smile that always got people to open up to him. He was liked by virtually everyone he met and touched.

Even when I was an infant, Dave watched over me. My first memory as a child is being six months old in a baby carriage outside our home at 37 Hawthorne Avenue. Yonkers was a hilly town and Hawthorne Avenue is a very steep street. It was Dave's hands I remember on the push bar. Dave would later tie rope, the kind that was used to wrap packages, to the carriage and let it roll down the hill to the very end of the length of the rope. It was a way of entertaining me. He thought I liked it.

For my part, I remember being terrified at the thought of not seeing hands on the push bar. A lot has been made over the years of the image of the terrified infant in the baby carriage with apparently no one holding on as I was rolling down the hill. Dave mistook my screams of fear for happiness.

The more I thought about it over the years and replayed the story in my head, the more I realize how comforting it was knowing that it was Dave on the other end of the rope, holding on to me, and that there was no way he would ever let go. Dave was always holding on to me — and I could always depend on him.

Dave had confidence in my artistic ability before anyone else did. Dave got me interested in music, then in comedy, and encouraged me to think creatively. He was the first person to cultivate my talent.

When you are starting out, nobody believes in you except, perhaps, close relatives and friends. You've got to believe in yourself, your ideas, and your talent, no matter what other people say. You must reject the negative instincts that drive the negative images (were they laughing at me or are they still laughing at the guy ahead of me?).

Until people know you're funny, they don't laugh. They think you're crazy. Your first test will be when you first walk out among strangers. You are going to get cotton mouth. You'll start to shake and start to sweat, and you haven't done anything yet. Then you push off into a monologue or a sketch. You do it with everything you've got and with control over your emotions, which is very hard. You need to understand the audience and how they are reacting to your comedy.

You can never fool the audience. They can always tell if you believe in yourself. Anytime I was in a show, Dave would send me a telegram to pump me up: "It's post time, Sid. Go get 'em. You've got to give it all you've got." The love and support that I got from Dave was as much a part of my success as anything else in my life. Dave knew.

My lifelong love of movies began as a child. The local Loews movie theater put a billboard up against the side of the building of my father's restaurant advertising their movies. In exchange, they would give my father two free tickets to the movies every week, usable only Monday through Friday. My father, mother, and Dave would take turns taking me to the movies.

In addition, I would go to the Saturday matinees religiously. As I got a little older, I was allowed to go alone. Once I went in at 10:00 a.m. and left at 6:00 p.m. I saw everything twice. A double feature, the newsreel, and a travelogue that emptied the theater. My father was worried because I was so late. When I finally came to the restaurant he was relieved that I was okay. He made me dinner, and as I ate he put his hand in his pocket as if he were going to give me money and said: "Would you like to go back for the evening performance?"

Dave took me to see the picture *Wings*. It was a silent movie about the flying corps in World War I. It was billed as "The Drama of the Skies — The war in the air from both sides of the lines." It was made in 1927 and was the first film to win the Oscar for Best Picture. Buddy Rogers and Richard Arlen fall for the same girl, Clara Bow, who was known as the "It Girl" (because she had "it" — sex appeal — in a time where you couldn't use the words "sex" or "pregnant"). After the United States enters World War I, both guys join the air corps and become aces. They remain friends, but their rivalry over the girl threatens their friendship. Dave and I ran home after the movie and couldn't stop talking about it.

We noticed that when the American guy got shot, there would only be a slight trickle of blood from his chin, and he would always be smiling, even when his plane spun out of control. But when the German pilot got shot, all hell broke loose. There was blood on the windshield, the cockpit was on fire, and there was smoke everywhere.

A few years later we saw *Test Pilot*, with Spencer Tracy and Clark Gable. Gable was the test pilot, and Tracy was the mechanic. And you knew right away if Gable didn't stick his little wad of gum at the back of the cockpit, you could take it to the bank that he wasn't coming back. If the gum was there, he'd be fine.

The star of the picture was the altitude meter. Gable goes over the top and then dives to test the plane. He goes higher and higher and then — VROOM — when the altitude meter reads three thousand feet he blacks out in the big crash dive! Our hearts were in our mouths as he falls toward the earth. The picture cuts to close-ups of people looking worried. But Gable makes it back safely, the gum still hanging on in the cockpit. He kisses the girl, shakes hands with his pal Spencer, and puts the gum back in his mouth. What a guy.

When I was seven years old, Dave and I wrote our first sketch together, about wartime airplane pictures and peacetime airplane pictures, which I would perform in front of the family on special occasions. In the wartime airplane pictures there was always a major in a little shack in an old bar with a dartboard and a couple of beer mugs. In our sketch, he's crying into his beer and slamming his fist on the bar, saying, "I should never have sent those men up in those crates with only a half hour's worth of training!" (Then he looks at the audience and says, "But it does save gas.") Then he hears the planes coming back and starts counting them. You hear the razzing sounds of the motors sputtering out (which I can't do anymore). When a plane crashes, the major says, "Okay, we've got four left."

In the part of the sketch about peace-time airplane movies, the pilot goes into the test dive. At three thousand feet, he passes out (and here we inserted more sputtering sounds). You see shots of the altitude meter, and shots of people screaming in horror as they watch the plane fall to certain doom. Three feet from the ground, he pulls the plane up to safety. He gets out, brushes himself off, kisses the girl, and walks away without so much as a scratch.

I also looked forward to Saturdays because I could listen to *Let's Pretend*, a very popular radio show at the time. I could see the princes and princesses, the castles and the villains in black armor in my mind's eye. As it did for many other children at the time, it got the creative juices flowing.

There was a record of Chinese music that my father had (I don't know why he bought it), that I would play over and over. I don't know why. To placate me, my father bought a piece of wax that was affixed to the arm of the Victrola (which you had to keep winding up to play) that would bring the needle back to the beginning each time the record ended. I would listen to the song in our living room, which had a rug with a design on it. As I would listen to the music, I would march around the perimeter of the rug. In my mind, the design of the rug went with the music. It was the beginnings of my use of music to help craft visual images.

I also listened to *The Make Believe Ballroom*, another very popular radio program, which was hosted by Martin Block. We had an old banjo in the house. I found two drumsticks, and I used to love to sit in the living room and play on the head of the banjo with the drumsticks. I would often wake Dave, who was sleeping during the day because he had worked the night shift. He never seemed to mind. He had enough trouble sleeping over the sounds of the new trolley tracks being put down.

Music was very important in my house growing up. My mother loved to play piano, and Abe and Dave both took piano lessons as well. My father was the only one who didn't play an instrument, but he loved music and had a collection of classical and opera recordings that I listened to. We listened to Cantor Yosele Rosenblatt singing "Kol Nidre" and "Eli, Eli" (which was a song to God), and Moishe Oysher, in addition to Georgie Jessel on the radio. (A favorite routine of his was a conversation with his mother: "Hello, Ma, this is your son. You know, from the money every week.")

To make up for his inability to give me more time and attention, my father did what most other immigrant Yonkers fathers did — he bought me things. One afternoon when I was nine years old I walked into the restaurant after school. "Sidney," my father said, "you're going to play the saxophone." "Why?" I asked. He was pointing to an old music case. "Because someone left one here. The cops said I could keep it if he didn't come back in thirty days. The thirty days are up, and it's yours."

My father also looked into music lessons for me. Once a week after school, I took the number 7 Yonkers trolley to the end of the line, and then rode a bus to the Hebrew National Home in Tuckahoe.

The music teacher was a genial man in his forties. Whenever I made a mistake, he would take my saxophone, put the mouthpiece between his own lips, and show me the phrasing of the piece, the way it should be played. When I had to play the passage again, I could taste whatever was on the lunch menu for the day: chopped liver, cabbage soup, or a little gedempte brust, which is roasted meat that had to be cooked a long time because it wasn't the best cut.

I probably would not have kept up with the saxophone if it weren't for Dave. Dave got me excited about music. When I got my saxophone, Dave spent $42 on a Conn tenor sax of his own, and we would play duets: "Two Tickets to Georgia," "Stars Fell on Alabama," and "I Found a Million Dollar Baby in a Five and Ten Cent Store." I started playing an alto sax and eventually played tenor sax. I also learned how to sight-read, which was tough.

Music became my first love. It also turned out to be great training because it gives you a sense of rhythm, timing, and discipline. You learn how to communicate in a different medium, which everyone can relate to and be touched by. In music, everyone phrases differently. It's not what you play; it's the way that you play it. You either feel the music or you don't. If it doesn't feel right, you know it's no good. Comedy works the same way.

I also took music appreciation classes in

school. When I was in the fifth grade, we had a class outing to the old Metropolitan Opera House in Manhattan. It was a defining experience for me. We got seats in the first few rows. I was more interested in the orchestra than I was in the singers. I studied the clarinet player closely because I was also studying clarinet at the time. Clarinet has almost the same fingering as the saxophone on one octave, but changes around the throat of the instrument.

The clarinet player didn't have much to do. He played a couple of notes, then rested for about half an hour. I was still fascinated. The arias were familiar to me because my father would play opera on the phonograph at home.

When I first started to play, I didn't enjoy the exercises because there were no tunes, just fingerings or, as they say, practice. When I got to play actual melodies it got very interesting. You wanted to play what you heard. The big sound of the day was syncopated New Orleans jazz. It was the first mainstream American music.

A new era was developing in music. You no longer had to stick to the same melodies and rhythms. Music got a lift. Composers like George Gershwin, Cole Porter, Victor Young, and lyricists like Oscar Hammerstein and Larry Hart took the music to the next level. They invented musical comedy. What the music did for me was not only train me as a musician, but also allow me to think creatively. You could ad-lib and be very creative as long as you stayed within the chord structure.

Comedy is music. It has a rhythm and a melody. It elicits passion, emotion, joy, and melancholy. And if you listen for it, you can hear a beat. I was very compulsive about practicing and getting my exercises and my phrasing right. When I was about fifteen, there was a certain interval I tried to get to, and each time I tried, I kept breaking up. I got so frustrated I put my fist into the living room wall. That didn't please my father one bit. It also didn't help my saxophone playing one bit. On top of that, I had to pay to repair the wall. I took my sax to a music shop and the guy there told me that the pads were leaking. He replaced the pads and I got the intervals on the first shot. It taught me a great lesson: It's not always you that's wrong.

The first inkling of music was really the drum. Just the drum. Then came the folk songs. The villagers would take a melody and put words to it. Then they added a few flutes and some stringed instruments. In the nineteenth century Franz Haydn, the father of the symphony, which was a series of melodies, brought together ten violins and formed an orchestra. Haydn was working for a royal family and had money to burn. He helped develop and evolve modern music.

The king and the prince were very fond of music, and Haydn would compose original pieces for them. Often the king would fall asleep while listening to the music. So Haydn wrote the *Surprise Symphony*. It starts off very soft and then graduates to the point where the cymbals and bass crash together. That would not only keep the king awake, but the shock sometimes required the chamber pot.

The classical era led to the Romantic composers, like Tchaikovsky and Rachmaninoff. Today, except for the movies, composers don't get the opportunity to develop grand compositions for large public consumption. Even then, it is rare that you get the kind of collaboration that exists between a Steven Spielberg and a John Williams and the majesty of the *Star Wars* theme.

Growing up, I had two heroes: Albert Einstein and the classical saxophonist Marcel Mule. I had a love for Einstein because of a love for science, particularly astronomy and physics, which began when I was a child. I love physics because I like to know how things work. I have always believed that there is an order and a rhythm to the world. God, as Einstein said, does not play dice with the universe. Things are ordered on our planet. There is a food chain. Elephants break down the forest and eat trees. The constant trampling of the herds of animals keeps the trees from growing, which results in meadow. The meadows allow other animal groups, like tigers and zebras, to flourish. The rhino grazes and the food becomes droppings. From the droppings of animals, you get forests again, and young animals thrive. When you lose the forest you lose everything.

When my son Rick was at Yale University, he left behind a physics textbook at home after a vacation. I picked it up, and for over thirty years I have been reading about physics. I am up to theories of gravity and the as yet unproven string theory.

Among musicians, I loved Marcel Mule because his music spoke to me. Mule was the greatest classical saxophonist in the world. He played with the Paris Conservatory, and I first heard him when I was a teenager. When Mule played Jacques Ibert's

Concertino da Camera, it was the first time I heard classical saxophone. Because the saxophone was a relatively new instrument, very little was written for it in symphonies — pieces were generally composed for more traditional woodwind instruments like the oboe, clarinet, flute, and English horn. I was so taken with the recording that I had to get my own copy of it.

A friend of mine wrote out the music for me from the recording, and I was able to study it. It was the first modern classical music that I liked. After that, my big dream was to go to Paris and study under Marcel Mule at the Paris Conservatory. World War II put that dream to bed.

My love of music also led me to appreciate the melodies and rhythms of foreign languages. I learned my signature double-talk, which was a fast-paced blend of different sounds and words mimicking French, Italian, German, Spanish, Russian, and other languages, from the customers at my father's restaurant. I went to school only a few blocks away and as soon as I was old enough, I used to clear tables and help my father out at lunchtime, which was the busiest time of day. I'd have my lunch and pick up some dishes. At night I would help Abe throw out the drunks who got a little too rowdy.

We had a night cashier, Jack, who was French. He taught me my first words in French: *Donnez-moi une tasse de café, s'il vous plaît:* Give me a cup of coffee, please. Dave worked the night shift with Jack, and Dave would imitate Jack for me. Watching Dave's imitation, I understood how he formed his lip movements and the intonations, and I was soon able to do it a little better. When I found I could do that, I learned that I could do it in German, Italian, and Russian.

Yonkers was a melting pot, a working-class town of immigrants from many countries who worked at the local factories and shops. Each of the different ethnic groups sat by themselves. Every time I'd go near a table, I would hear the distinct language and pick up some words and sounds, which were often curse words, which I knew never to use.

I would go from table to table, listening to the sounds. I would hear the groups speak Italian, Russian, Polish, Hungarian, French, Spanish, Lithuanian, and even Bulgarian. I would pick up words and the nuances of the dialects and the tones, and would speak to them in double-talk, which was as close as I came to actually learning the language. The first time I tried it out was in front of a table of Italians. I was so young, my head barely reached above the table. When I rattled away in fake Italian, they listened to me and smiled, certain I was one of their own. Then they tried to figure out what I was saying, and quickly realized I was speaking gibberish. They loved it.

The Italians sent me over to a table of Poles to do the same routine in Polish. Pretty soon I had the entire restaurant laughing; I had found my way into a comic device that became one of my trademarks. (Though I didn't know it, an earlier vaudeville comic, Willie Howard, had been doing double-talk in Yiddish for years.)

Every language has its own song and its own rhythm. In order to do double-talk, you think in English and say the words like they have a purpose. It's the nuances and the inflections that make the audience believe that you are actually speaking the language you are double-talking in. Japanese is guttural, like German. Chinese is more melodic. There are so many different dialects that people in one town can't understand the people in the next one over the hill. To this day, people are shocked when they learn that English is the only language I speak, and even that not too fluently.

What was also important about my new-found gift was that I could make my parents laugh and hold their attention, too. Dave and I used to get a lot of laughs in the family parlor doing double-talk.

I would even do double-talk in synagogue. I wasn't doing it disrespectfully, but out of a desire to fit in and impress. There seemed to be a race to finish the prayers among the synagogue elders, which would end with the winner closing the prayer book shut while holding it up in the air. The double-talk made it seem like I was moving through the prayer book like a Torah scholar, as I would also slam the prayer book shut. The synagogue elders were in awe over my apparent expertise in the Scripture.

Years later, when *Your Show of Shows* became a hit, I was brought up to the Waldorf Towers to meet General Dwight D. Eisenhower. Ike had sat in on many conferences with Russian generals. "I heard you can do something in Russian," he said. "Da," I replied, and lapsed into Russian double-talk. "That's exactly how they sound," he told me. Another time I spoke in Chinese double-talk and a columnist, Frank Farrell, who as a marine had been stationed in the Far East, asked me if the dialect wasn't from the north of China.

Later, when we did parodies of foreign movies every week on *Your Show of Shows*, Carl Reiner, Mel Brooks, and I would go out with our wives on a theme night. If we did a French foreign movie, we'd go to a French restaurant. If a German restaurant was hard to find, we'd go to a Jewish restaurant. We found a lot of material there.

For years, anytime Florence and I were abroad, I would order the food in double-talk or call over the maître d' and just strike up a conversation. In Rome, I said, "Florence, I'm going to order in Italian." Florence would get embarrassed. "Don't start," she warned, "we'll get in trouble." "No," I said, "it will be all right." I would do my double-talk and the waiter would watch my finger on the menu and know what we wanted to order. I think I have caused a few waiters to order psychiatrists.

If you get a break, it means that fate has dealt you a good card. There is such a thing as luck. There absolutely is. It often comes when you least expect it. That's why you should always be prepared for it. If you throw a million quarters in the air, half of them will likely land heads and the other half tails. Eighty or ninety in a row may land heads. That's a run of luck. But you have to be prepared for that luck.

Just having been given the gift of double-talk could be called luck. Putting it to use in the foreign movies that we did is taking it to the next level, and good things happened. If you believe in yourself and work hard, you will be prepared when your break comes. You can help fate and make the break work, with preparation, dedication, and passion. If you're not prepared, no amount of luck will get you to the next level.

I didn't know how I was able to do the double-talk and I don't want to know how. Never look a gift horse in the mouth. And if it ain't broke, don't fix it. People with no real background or ability will always try and tell you how to improve your skills. I always think about the story I heard about Yehudi Menuhin in this respect. Menuhin, the son of Russian immigrants, was a child prodigy violinist who was a few years older than I was. Menuhin first heard classical music as a toddler when his parents took him to concerts to avoid paying for a baby-sitter. He gave his first concert at the tender age of seven. I heard it told that all the greatest violin teachers came to the performance. Yehudi played and he was fantastic. There was a standing ovation, and everyone was raving. After the concert the great master teachers came backstage to visit him and each one said the same thing — it's not only that you have the technique, but to play with such soul at the age of seven and with such phrasing, it's a miracle.

The last teacher came over to him and said, "You're wonderful. You're a genius. You really are. You play the violin like you own it. But, if I may make one tiny observation, when you get into the harmonics, you tend to be a little . . . *sharp.*" For the first time in his life, Yehudi looked down at his fingers and he had to learn to play the violin all over again. All over again. All because of one jerk, who thought the performance was a little sharp. He had to find something. A genius compromised.

One of the reasons I never questioned good luck when it came was because I knew what bad luck was. I was seven when the Great Depression struck in 1929, and it hit our family hard. Before the stock market crashed, my family was very comfortable financially. My father also invested in real estate and owned property and apartment buildings in both New York and Florida. After the crash, my father began to lose everything. I watched the toll this took on both my parents, particularly my father, and it had a big impact on me.

The family eventually moved out of the house on 37 Hawthorne Avenue into six small rooms over the restaurant. Because of my constant practicing on the saxophone there was a switch in the popularity of the other sixty-nine rooms that were still being rented out to guests. The fifty cents a night inner rooms without the windows were now more popular than the seventy-five cents a night windowed rooms, because it was harder for the sound of the saxophone to penetrate the walls. I made a deal with the guy who lived upstairs that I wouldn't start practicing until after 5:00 p.m.

I remember eating a lot of cereal with hot water and potatoes with sour cream. We learned not to make demands. If you wanted to go to the movies, you collected bottles and turned them in for two cents apiece. And to this day, I have never played the stock market. I always bought insured bonds. You know the rate of return you're going to get, you get your money back, and you don't have to worry whether the market goes up or down.

Despite the Depression, my father took us out whenever he could. It was important to him. We would take a day's excursion into New York City, to the Lower East

Side. There were no expressways yet, so we traveled through the hilly streets of Yonkers, down Broadway from Washington Heights to midtown Manhattan, and then down Park Avenue until we hit Hester Street. We would drop my mother off before 1:00 p.m. so that she could get into the Roxy Theater for a quarter.

After the movies my mother would go shopping. She would start out in one shop and emerge from another shop a block away and across the street. There was an underground labyrinth of tunnels connecting the stores that she never talked about.

While my mother was at the movies, my father and I went to the Russian steam baths on St. Mark's Place. Sitting in the *shvitz*, as it was called in Yiddish, I was told that one of the rites of passage to manhood was being able to withstand the heat on the top shelf closest to where the steam was released, turning over only four times. I was nowhere near being able to accomplish such a task at my young age.

My mother would meet us at the baths, and we would have dinner at Rattners, Moskowitz & Lupowitz, or some other restaurant, where two and a half dollars could feed the whole family. When you sat at a table, you would get a "blue bottle" of seltzer. Seltzer was also known as "two cents plain." I remember an egg cream was a nickel. There was also a drink called an "eingemach," which was a concoction of all of the syrups, cherry, chocolate, and pineapple that would drip away into the small basin below the soda fountain captured in small glasses and would then be resurrected into a new drink that cost three cents. You could either have an eingemach or a Charlotte Russe. To have both would have been considered excessive.

My mother would talk about the vast acquisitions she made at bargain prices. My father would be in an unusually mellow mood and would talk about his early days in the United States. Dinner would be followed by a walk around Houston Street, not far from where my father grew up.

We spent the summers during those years in Rockaway Beach, New York. The family stayed in one room that cost $125 for the entire summer, which ran from the beginning of June to the end of October.

I looked forward to Yom Kippur every year. It was my Christmas. I got a new suit, new shoes, and new socks. I wore knickers until after my bar mitzvah. Long pants for me were a big deal. It meant manhood. I was so excited that I threw up when carrying my suit home.

Yom Kippur always coincided with the World Series. One year, I was excused from the service at the Agudath Achim Synagogue during Yizkor, the portion where the survivors mourn their dead. I wandered over to Herald Square, where the *Yonkers Herald-Statesman* had a huge electric board, which gave a play-by-play of the action between the Philadelphia Athletics and the St. Louis Cardinals. I became so involved in the game that I lost track of time and was a half hour late getting back to shul. My father took me outside. "Where'd you go?" he asked. "I was following the game and I lost track of time," I told him. "Would you like to go back there and check the score?" As I said no, bam! He smacked me.

When I was eleven years old, Dave took me down to the Savoy Ballroom in Manhattan. Drummer Chic Webb was leading the orchestra and Ella Fitzgerald was singing. She was a great jazz vocalist who introduced a whole new style of singing, and she was also from Yonkers. She was only sixteen years old at the time. I remember how great she looked and how great she sounded. I also saw Lester Young playing with Count Basie. Lester was one of the first modern jazz saxophone players. I was probably too young to be taken out to the city at night, but Dave knew how important it would be for me and how much I would enjoy it.

Dave and I went to the Savoy Ballroom one year on *erev* Rosh Hashanah, the night before the Jewish New Year. We got back at four in the morning and we had to be in synagogue at 8:30. Eight-thirty came and my father was already in synagogue with Abe.

To say that my father was angry was an understatement. He had spent $50 for tickets for the family and he expected us to be there with him on the high holidays. My father went back home to find us. We had a sliding door in our house. I remember my father coming up the stairs and then the sliding door opening. Dave was already six feet two and 260 pounds, but he was still having trouble holding off my enraged father with one hand and getting dressed with the other. I got dressed quickly and was out of the house before my father could grab me.

Like almost every other Jewish kid in the world, I went to afternoon Hebrew school from the age of five until I was bar mitzvahed at age thirteen. Like most kids, I found Hebrew school a tedious experience. It was a long time to be watching the clock in sheer boredom. I remember drawing pictures of the teacher as Frankenstein with a little arrow pointing to a note that read: "Notice the pipe in his neck."

My father somehow found the money for the bar mitzvah lessons and for my bar mitzvah in 1935. It was the height of the Depression, but my father still made a party for me. When I realized how much it meant to him, it made my becoming a man under Jewish law all the more important and poignant. I made a speech about how grateful I was to my family for not skipping this important day in my life, which other families did to save money. There wasn't a dry eye in the house. My speech even brought tears to the rabbi's eyes.

As the oldest brother, Abe took the brunt of my father's toughness. A woman who worked as a telephone operator would come into the restaurant regularly. Abe fell in love and wanted to marry her. She wasn't Jewish, and my father said, "If you marry her, you have to leave the house." There was no other work to be had during the Depression, and Abe reluctantly acquiesced. His heart was broken and he never married after that. He was afraid to.

My father went bankrupt in 1935. He not only lost the St. Claire Buffet and Luncheonette but also some real estate he had owned in Yonkers and Florida. He looked around and found a luncheonette on Chambers Street in Manhattan. He commuted every day, taking the trolley to Van Cortlandt Park, followed by the train to Chambers Street, which was almost the end of the line — over two hours each way. In time, he lost the Chambers Street business, and then ran the small Main Lunch Bar back in Yonkers, two doors down from the St. Claire Buffet, and lost that as well. He also opened a novelty shop on Manor House Square in Yonkers and worked there with Dave. One Halloween day, they took in over $100 selling magnetic dogs whose heads spun around and fake dog turds.

When I finished P.S. 10 elementary school, I entered Benjamin Franklin Junior High School, which was in the Italian section of town. No day at Benjamin Franklin Junior High was complete without a fistfight at the end of the day. Fighting was almost an extracurricular activity. Because I was one of the bigger kids, I was expected to lead the battles. Every afternoon I left school and waited for the other kids to get out, always keeping my back to the wall. I would take off my coat and say, "Let's go." As soon as the three o'clock bell sounded, it was — bang! — a fight. I hit people and I got hit. I learned to always keep myself in good shape and prepared.

Finally my mother petitioned the board of education and got me transferred to Nathaniel Hawthorne Junior High. It was a very high-class school. There was only one fight a week.

The fighting aside, I grew up in a time of innocence. People put aspirin in Coca-Cola because they thought it made them high. We didn't know about the harmful effects of the sun. People used to put iodine on and sunbathe to get a rich tan. We didn't hear about marijuana or cocaine. I first saw marijuana when I was a professional musician. I turned it down because it was illegal. Drinking, however, was legal, and I began as a young man.

I generally liked school. I rarely needed to do any homework because I paid attention in class. I developed the ability to memorize what I heard early on. The less homework I needed to do, the more I could practice my music. That ability to understand what

I heard helped me memorize lines and dialogue quickly in later years. Junior high and high school were all about music for me. When I think of my high school experiences, I think of Woody Allen's movie *Radio Days*, in which the setting and all of the songs come so close to capturing the warmth of the time and my experiences. I especially liked the scene where the beautiful substitute teacher walks into the classroom and just mesmerizes the room. That happened to us many times.

I also remember walking into Radio City for the first time. It was like walking onto a Hollywood set. I remember looking around in awe, stunned by its beauty. The architecture, color, the staircase, chandeliers, and the great stage. There wasn't a pole in the place. After all these years, it still has the same grandeur and majesty. Little did I know that a few years later I would be playing in the great hall's sister theater, the Center Theater, which was across the street.

I have always been fascinated by history. The background of a lot of comedy is history. If you study how people walked, how they acted, how they negotiated with each other, how they adopted status symbols in certain periods, you have the basis of a lot of good funny sketches.

I had this fantasy that I was a direct descendant of Julius Caesar. "It just might be," I thought to myself. I carefully studied all about Roman history, the Gallic wars, the invasion of England, everything.

Years later Florence and I went to Rome with another couple. "Why don't we hire a guide?" I said. "It'll only cost a couple of bucks and we'll know what we're looking at." So we ordered a guide. The man that was sent to us showed us all kinds of credentials and badges all over the place. He started to take us around.

"This here is the place where they buried Julius Caesar," he said.

I looked at him. "No one knows where Julius Caesar is buried."

He pointed at the badge on his coat. "You see this?" he said, "Official guide. It's from the government."

He took us to another location. "Now over here," he said, "this is the place where Marc Antony made the speech for Julius Caesar."

I looked at him again. "Marc Antony never made a speech for Julius Caesar. It's only in the play."

"You see what I got here?" he said, pointing to his badges again. "That's from the government."

His confidence not shaken one bit by my corrections, he took us to another location. "You see over there? That's the Palatine Hill. The palace of Augustus Caesar was there. And over here was the palace of Octavian."

"No, no," I said. "Augustus Caesar and Octavian Caesar were the same person. Octavian took the name of Augustus Caesar."

He looked at me. "What do you think, you know history? What's your name?"

"Caesar," I told him.

"You?"

"Sidney Caesar," I said. "Here's my passport."

"Oh, no wonder you know," he said.

By the time I got to Yonkers High School I was already six feet tall, which made the football coach drool over me every day like I was a piece of fresh meat. "Left tackle," he would say to me. I told him that I wasn't going to play ball because I couldn't afford to hurt my lips, because then I couldn't play the sax. "Don't worry," the coach told me. "We'll fix you up with protective gear so nothing will happen to your lips."

The coach was both persistent and reassuring. I gave in and decided to give

66

football a try. I spent hours with the team trainer, working with wire protective devices, adhesive tape, and masks. I put on the uniform, shoulder pads, and the old-fashioned leather helmets. Facemasks hadn't been invented yet.

I jogged out onto the field like a gridiron hero from the movies. During the first scrimmage — bang! Bloody nose and split lip. I took off the helmet and uniform and the lip guard and gave it to the coach. "If this doesn't heal it's gonna cost you three bucks," I said, and walked off the field.

The split lip soon healed and I joined a group called Mike Cifficello's Swingtime Six. Mike played the piano. Saul Rosenbaum played alto sax (I played tenor sax). Tony Cacciatore played the trumpet and Al De Famio was our drummer. We played at school and Italian weddings, which were also known as "football weddings" because of the small wrapped sandwiches that were tossed at the guests like little footballs. We also played at restaurants and bars all over Yonkers, including the Polish Community Center. These were the kinds of joints with signs outside that read: "Dining, Dancing, and Fighting."

Often I would be invited to Sunday dinner by one of the Italian band members.

I loaded up on spaghetti because I thought that's all there was to eat; I didn't know that it was just the appetizer. Then came the chicken, the fish, and the meat (and then the bathroom). It was a time and a culture where you couldn't not eat. If it was put on your plate, you ate it.

We memorized "The Star Spangled Banner" immediately. As soon as we heard someone say "Hey, you stink," which was invariably followed by "Oh, yeah!" in Italian, Russian, German, Hungarian, Polish, Lithuanian, or even Bulgarian, it was a cue to stop whatever we were playing at the time, play the National Anthem, and bring everyone to attention. Sometimes it worked, sometimes it didn't.

Those gigs paid between two and three dollars a man. Since my father had lost the restaurant, I "gave to the house," as it was then called. I gave $2.50 to my father and kept fifty cents for myself, which paid for the movies. Once we played at a basketball game and had to split a buck and a half between six people. We used the money to buy more orchestrations and build our library.

We got a New Year's Eve gig with a contract that called for us to play from 9:00 p.m. "until unconscious," or until the last drunk got thrown out. We also had to wear tuxedos. I borrowed Abe's blue suit, got a vest, and bought a bow tie at Woolworth's for ten cents.

When I got a bit older, I'd blow fifty cents on a date. Two seats in the balcony for a picture, and two sodas after that. Home late at the time meant eleven o'clock. It was the height of luxury if your family had a car and you got to take your date out that way. I don't remember having many dates in high school. On one date, I had to pay fifty cents for each of us for a dance and ten cents each for sodas. I wanted to walk her home, not for the romantic component but because I wanted to save ten cents on the trolley.

I graduated Yonkers High School in June of 1939. I was sixteen and was at a crossroads. The Depression had taken an emotional toll on my father. I wasn't bringing enough money into the house and they couldn't afford to keep me. I needed to be on my own, and I needed to help out.

I knew about the American Federation of Musicians in New York City. I heard that a good saxophone player could make as much as $40 a week. With that in mind, I headed south to Manhattan.

The people at Local 802 of the musician's

union were very nice to me. They thought I was at least twenty. They said I couldn't become a member until I had lived in the city for six months and established residency.

I went to my father's brother, my Uncle Joe, in Manhattan. He ran a hotel with rooms that cost fifty cents a night, and he took me in for free. I remember looking out the window at the Empire State Building and thinking, "New York. This will be a tough town to beat." I didn't even have ten cents in my pocket.

Chapter 2

FROM SAX TO COMEDY

In many ways my life began in the Catskills Mountains in upstate New York, because of two things that happened to me. The first was I learned I could make audiences laugh on a consistent basis; I could develop sketches. The second, and more important, was that it was up there that I met Florence, the love of my life for over sixty years.

Artists come in clusters during any period of time. Haydn and Beethoven were contemporaries. So were Monet and Renoir. Paris was a locus of artists at the turn of the nineteenth century. The Impressionist painters, such as Renoir, Monet, Pissarro, and Morisot, weren't considered real artists at the time because their styles were so new and radical. Their work was rejected by the Salon, a juried art exhibition sponsored annually by the official French Academy of Fine Arts. It was put on exhibit for the first time at a studio in Paris in 1874. They

71

were the outcasts, they painted outside the lines. But they would all get together at night at cheap restaurants in Paris and would drink together and discuss each other's styles.

What late-nineteenth-century Paris was to art, mid-twentieth-century America was to comedy. And one of the centers of that creativity was the Catskill Mountains resorts in upstate New York.

In the late 1930s and 1940s, the Catskill Mountains were college for many entertainers, myself included. In the hundreds of resorts, hotels, and bungalow colonies, the audiences were tough and demanded quality. The Catskills created a Jewish *Brigadoon* and provided a training ground for young comedians and musicians.

People went to the Catskills in droves from New York City and stayed at least a week. The top customer paid $35 a week. The average hotel had two hundred rooms, ten meals a day — at least it seemed like ten — and all the sour cream, buttermilk, and green chicken you could stand. There was a little casino and a small social staff. There were no headliners or big celebrities. If you were there for the summer, you were there for ten weeks.

By way of context, at my father's restaurant

breakfast — three eggs any style, toast, and coffee — was fifteen cents. Milk was twelve cents a quart. A loaf of bread was five or six cents. If you were making $50 a week in those days, you were thinking about marriage.

If you were spending a week's salary on a hotel stay, you expected to eat. You actually overate because you wanted to get your money's worth. The dining room was all about more. "Bring me another chocolate. Make it two. No, make it three. Okay — we'll all have it, what the hell."

There was a walking area outside that everyone went to after meals, which was for conversation, great or otherwise. The "bull" train used to come in on Friday night. That's when, as the joke went, the husbands showed up and all the waiters had to move out. The normal things that go on in regular life went on in the Catskills. The culture and the environment were just freer.

It was a wonderful era. It was very edifying because you met so many different kinds of people, a lot of them educated and knowledgeable. There were philosophical discussions with arguments on the lawn that went far into the night. It was a very cultural environment, like a kibbutz with a lot of food.

Burlesque was in full bloom then, but the burlesque houses would close during the summer because they had no air-conditioning. So the burlesque performers would go up to the mountains for ten weeks and make a hundred bucks. It was a big change for them, going from their risqué world to performing in front of audiences that wouldn't let you use the word "damn."

I was fourteen when I first went up to the Catskills as a musician. During my sophomore year in high school, while I was playing with Mike Cifficello's Swingtime Six, Mike booked us at the Anderson Hotel in Monticello, New York. In addition to our five-piece band, there was a comic, a dancer, and a singer. The master of ceremonies was also the straight man. They would also do little sketches. One day we were rehearsing and the comedian, Jackie Michaels, the house comic, was looking for cheap help and was asking for volunteers to be in the show. "Yeah," I said, "I'll help you." I was always eager to be in show business.

Jackie, whose training was in burlesque, wanted me to be in a mind-reading sketch. "We're gonna blindfold you, ask you one question and that's it," he said. "Sure," I said. "I can do that." I put on my one good suit. I put on a tie. I got a shirt all cleaned and pressed and my shoes shined. I was very excited about being onstage.

Capacity was about ninety people. At a hundred the room was jammed. I went onstage and they blindfolded me. Jackie asked, "What is this? What do I have in my hand — an egg or a tomato?" I answered, "An egg." "Wrong, a tomato!" he said, smashing the tomato in my face.

It got a big laugh from the audience. I took the blindfold off. I looked down. There was tomato all over my face and my suit. I was stunned, surprised, and pissed off. I had just one suit, I was wearing it, and it was now garnished with tomato. I yelled, "What are you doing?" I looked him straight in the eye, and he knew I was coming for him. As I made my move toward him, Jackie jumped off the stage and I took off after him. The audience was screaming with laughter.

I finally caught Jackie when he stopped running. He was out of breath but still smiling. He apologized and asked me not to hit him. "You're the first laugh I ever got working clean," he said.

"Who's gonna pay for the suit?" I asked. He said, "I'll have it cleaned for you. And if you'd like, you can help out once in a while on the stage." The boss came over and said, "If you help Jackie, you don't have to play during lunch, and I'll give you another dollar a week." I was now making $10 a week and I was getting my suit cleaned for free. I knew I was on my way.

The summer of 1939, after I graduated from high school, I got another summer job playing the saxophone at the Vacationland Hotel in Swan Lake, which was also in the Catskills. There I met another one of my great influences, Don Appel, the social director. The social director's role was very important in the Catskill hotels. When the hotel hired him in the spring, he was responsible for hiring staff, which generally consisted of the usual comic, straight man, singer, and dancer. The social director was master of ceremonies, in charge of assembling the entertainment staff and running all of the programs. He was also a promoter, responsible for keeping the guests occupied and making friends with each other. This was done during the day with organized games and at night in the hotel's theater, which was known as the casino, pronounced "casina." If it rained, there was dancing in the casino.

The band was hired separately by the

hotel, so I wasn't part of the social staff. But I still offered to help out with the shows. I was a musician who stood in as a comic. Don was grateful for the free help and let me work part-time.

Don at the time was in his late twenties. His ambition was to do theater, and he later produced plays on Broadway for the legendary Yiddish comedienne, Molly Picon. One of his neighbors and protégés was a young Melvin Kaminsky, who grew up to be Mel Brooks, who was only thirteen at the time. Mel was a drummer who worked as a tummler, someone who entertained the guests at the pool or in the lobby of the hotel and got them to participate in activities. He was a crazy, loud teenager, always animated and very funny. He would do a routine where he would dress as a businessman in a suit and overcoat, carrying suitcases. At poolside, he would say, "Is this where you check in?" and walk off the diving board into the pool, fully clothed.

Don Appel was a good professor, a great introduction to show business. We did full shows, including *Pins and Needles*, about the needle workers union, *Carousel*, *The Monkey's Paw*, *Golden Boy*, and *Waiting for Lefty*. That socially conscious Clifford Odets play had one of my favorite lines.

The father comes back from visiting his son's apartment and tells his wife, "Mama, you should've seen. He had pajamas — satin — $50 a pair! And a toilet like a monument!"

It was there at Vacationland that I learned to act and perform comedy. The schedule was the same all over the Catskills. Monday night was bingo night (the only night we performers had off), Tuesdays was dancing. Wednesday was the small revue. Thursday was game night. Friday nights were plays and on Saturday night there was the full revue. Sunday night was guest night, comedy and amateur night — anybody could get up and sing and dance. New guests would check in on Sunday night and were able to meet and greet each other.

I did three shows a week. There was a new show every week in two- to three-week cycles, because that's how long each guest usually stayed. It didn't feel like work for me because I could memorize lines very quickly by just looking at the page. It was a great school and an amazing education.

Every summer, as the comedians arrived at the hotels, they would open an old trunk and take out even older material. Formula routines had names like "Little Joe" and

"Dirty Socks." I thought that the routines and the shtick that was being used to entertain were familiar and tired. People knew the routines by heart and were just waiting for the punch line. It was there, in an attempt to do something new, that I first started developing sketch comedy. I knew one simple fact: Two people sitting at a table was a sketch. I also knew from entertaining the customers at my father's restaurant that there was humor in the little things that people did. If you showed them how they looked when they did what they did, they would laugh.

I told Don, "There is something funny about two guys going to the *shvitz* (the steam room)."

"What's funny about it?" he asked.

"The way you walk in," I said. "You immediately duck because of the blast of heat. You start talking about how hot it is. 'It's hot, oh boy is it hot. You think it'll get hotter? I hope so. Throw another bucket on the coals, but tell me before you do it, because that's some breeze!'"

We did the sketch and people laughed. They had never seen themselves parodied before. I give Don a lot of credit for letting me run with the ideas. After all, I was just a kid.

I wanted to extend the sketches. Don was initially reluctant but after some thought was willing to try. So I got to work. Two guys in the *shvitz* in a contest of wills, putting pail after pail of water on the hot rocks, to see who can last the longest. ("You think this is hot, I'll show you hot! You're starting to turn red!" "It's not hot enough." "It's hot enough." "Well it's hot enough for me." "Do you want to stay here?" "I'm going to put another pail in." "Don't put another pail in, because if you put another pail in I'm going to be hot"). Two guys in a bakery, shopping for challah. I even worked in some of my double-talk in different languages. Some bits worked better than others, but people were coming over from other hotels to see our improvisations. At the time, fifty people was a big draw. The Catskill audiences were tough. Some of them didn't laugh at anything.

It was the first time I really learned how to play with an audience. I knew that by giving them what they knew I could entertain them. It was also the first time I began to realize that I could make things up myself, which was a wonderful realization for an entertainer.

A lot of the humor was an outgrowth of

the misunderstandings between Yiddish and English and the melding of European and American cultures. For instance, I knew someone who worked as a busboy. He was a very big and affable guy. He could carry tremendous amounts of dishes. But he had trouble understanding the clientele. An old woman called him over and said, "Bring me a bekked teppel." *Teppel* is the Yiddish for bowl or ladle, so he brought out one of those big ladles. She looked at the ladle and yelled, "I wanted a bekked teppel!" Somehow the volume made the language clearer. "Oh, you want a baked apple!" the busboy said. "Why didn't you say so?"

After two summers in Vacationland, Don moved the troupe to Kutsher's Country Club in Monticello. It was one of the premier hotels in the Catskills, and is one of only four establishments that are still operating. There my roles were reversed. I was now a full-time comedian and a stand-in musician, who occasionally helped out in the band. We were now developing a trunkful of new sketches, so many that we didn't use one old routine the entire season.

The management didn't understand what I was doing. I didn't tell jokes. I did funny bits. They didn't understand why they were paying a young kid who didn't tell jokes as a comedian. They were looking for a tummler, someone like Mel Brooks, a person who was the life of the party, who was less a performer and more of a live wire who jumped around as a catalyst to encourage guests to become involved in activities. The word came down that I was going to be fired.

The night before I was supposed to leave, I did a sketch called "The Crazy House." I played an inmate in a lunatic asylum who was trying to escape. Two other guys played the asylum guards who tried to catch me. I kept breaking free of their grasp. I was running through the audience, yelling and throwing rolls of toilet paper into the air. I was doing improvisational comedy onstage. The audience loved it. The management had never seen an audience react quite that enthusiastically.

The sketch and I were the big topic of conversation at breakfast the following morning. My bags were already packed and I was waiting for the hotel bus to take me back to Monticello and then to catch the bus to New York City, when the manager came over. "Let's not be hasty," he said. "I think we have a place for you."

During the summer of 1942, Don moved

the troupe yet again, to the Avon Lodge in Woodridge, New York. The Avon Lodge was owned by a man named Meyer Arkin. Meyer had a niece named Florence Levy, who was working that summer as a hotel governess.

The very first time I saw Florence, it was through an office window in a walkway between two buildings. It was like a frame. She was tall and willowy, and had silky pale blond hair pulled back over perfect features and the brightest, biggest blue-gray eyes. I had never seen anyone so beautiful in my life. I had seen showgirls and singers before, but never anyone like her. Her intelligent and ladylike movements radiated class. I was smitten.

I was only nineteen but I remember thinking, "That's the girl I'm going to marry." I went right over to her and said hello. I uncharacteristically told her, "I have absolutely fallen in love."

Florence had made a date with some other guy before she met me, and he came up to see her, which made me furious. It was like I was married to her already. I am still mad over it.

I began my campaign right away. I used to see her every day. It was the perfect place to court a young woman. There was a pool, a lake with rowboats — it was all very romantic. We didn't go anywhere, but we would just take walks along the road and get a soda. You didn't do anything in those days. You were lucky if you got a kiss. But when you did it was amazing. If you got to put your arm around your girl, wow!

Florence was a student at Hunter College at the time. She was not just beautiful; she had a good mind and a great conception of everything. Florence introduced me to art and culture. I was rough and unpolished, used to fighting for everything I got. But I did know something about music, current events, world history. I regaled Florence with my knowledge of politics and great battles. We would take long walks and have even longer discussions about art, politics, and history. I wanted to learn new things, particularly art, but didn't know how to go about it. Florence introduced me to new ideas. Florence had a very calming effect on me. When she wasn't with me I was like a tiger. She made me want to be smart and become the best version of myself. She brought out the best side of me.

Florence bought me the first book about art that I ever read in its entirety — *Lust for Life* by Irving Stone, about the life of Vincent van Gogh. Van Gogh was a violent, clumsy, passionate man who was driven to exhaustion and ultimately insanity by his fervor to put the essence of life into his art. I always identified with the artist who gave all of himself for his art.

We were married a little over a year later. Many people who met up there got married. Probably 60 percent of Jewish marriages in New York and New Jersey at the time were between people who met in the mountains. I am lucky to have been one of those people.

Chapter 3

THE SUBWAY COMMANDOS

I was trying to get into the musician's union, the Local 802, and had to establish residency in Manhattan for six months before I could play as a union member. I had been looking for a job as an usher. My first stop was the Roxy Theater. The atmosphere was cold, antiseptic, and regimented. It felt like West Point. Everyone who worked there wore white gloves. I had to fill out all kinds of forms. When I got to the question that asked for my religion, I wrote "purple."

I then went to Manhattan's Capitol Theatre, on Broadway between 50th and 51st Streets. It was in the upper part of the theater district, where the application process was a little simpler. I walked into the office and said, "I'm looking for a job as an usher." They looked at me and said, "You got it." I wore a forty-four coat top and a thirty-four bottom. They had to break up a set to make my uniform.

My first job there was standing in aisle 4, saying, "This way." Not very demanding. The Capitol was a very fancy theater and showed only first-run MGM movies. The first picture I ushered at was *Boom Town*, with Clark Gable, Spencer Tracy, and Lana Turner. I saw that picture many, many times. I amused myself by reciting the dialogue under my breath in the darkened theater.

Then one day the manager, Mr. Pearlman, said, "Sidney, how would you like to make $18 a week instead of $15? You've got a good physique; how would you like to be a doorman?" In actuality, the doorman quit because winter was coming up, and no one else could fit into the uniform. It was $3 more a week, so I wasn't complaining. Plus, I would often get 10¢ tips for opening the door, which I was supposed to do anyway. Occasionally an MGM movie star like Lana Turner or Claire Trevor would show up for an opening. I was assigned to escort the star to the elevator, so her shoes would not get dirty walking up the stairs, and take her to the loge seats, which were $1.25. Could you imagine standing next to Lana Turner in an elevator?

As I walked my post on Broadway, I was already working out comedy routines in my head. A couple once approached me and asked, "Do we have time for a sandwich before the show starts?" "That depends on what kind of sandwich you want, a fast sandwich or a slow sandwich," I told them. "A fast sandwich is bacon and tomato, where the bacon is already made up. A slow sandwich is like pastrami, where you wait around for them to slice the meat. If you have it toasted, it will add another five minutes." I would glance at my watch for effect. "You couldn't get away with anything slower than egg salad or tuna fish," I concluded, touching my fingers to my cap. They thanked me and gave me a dime tip.

On the coldest days of the year Dave drove my mother down from Yonkers to the theater. I would move the stanchions out from the no parking zone, so he could park in front of the marquee. My mother would get out of the car and give me homemade tomato soup in a thermos and a warm dickey, like the cops would wear, to put around my neck. At the time I didn't realize how lucky I was to have both a mother and a brother of that caliber.

On Sunday afternoon, December 7, 1941, I was walking up and down in front of the theater. You weren't allowed to "bark" (which was yelling, "Now playing at the theater is . . ."). You also weren't allowed to talk to anyone, unless the other person approached you first, and even then it was sotto voce.

All of a sudden soldiers, sailors, and marines started running out of the theater. I thought the place was on fire! Then I realized that only servicemen were running. I looked down Broadway, and I could see a corner of the Times Building, which had the revolving news ticker. It said, BATTLE-SHIP ARIZONA SUNK . . . PACIFIC FLEET . . . SEVEN SHIPS SUNK. I felt a rush of fear and excitement. I kept hearing the words "here we go" in my head over and over. I knew my life had changed at that moment.

Up to then I had been living in a rooming house run by a Mrs. Fuchs, who was a housemother for aspiring musicians. It was on 50th Street and Eighth Avenue, across the street from the old Madison Square Garden. Breakfast was twenty-five cents, dinner was thirty-five. For a buck a day you could live well. I had a little radio I would listen to. Henry Morgan was one of my favorites. I would also go to the automat and make tomato soup out of the free boiling water and the free catsup. Not nearly as good as my mother's.

During the breaks from my job at the

Capitol Theatre, I studied with Frank Chase of the NBC Symphony. He had played the clarinet, oboe, flute, bassoon, and saxophone for Arturo Toscanini and Andre Kostelanetz. He gave lessons from a little studio at 50th Street and Sixth Avenue. "Your tone is the best thing about you," he would tell me. He was an excellent teacher who lived well into his nineties.

I also studied at the Juilliard School of Music in Manhattan, though I was never formally registered. I went in and played the saxophone and the clarinet for the admissions director. "You're a musician," he told me, and I was allowed to audit classes. I got some pencils, bought the books, and sat in. I studied harmony, theory, and orchestration for six months.

After I joined the musicians union in 1942, one of the other musicians at Mrs. Fuchs's rooming house was impressed with my playing and got me a booking with Shep Field's orchestra, which at the time consisted of nine saxophones outside the rhythm section. My days as a movie doorman were over.

I spent only two weeks with Shep Field and his orchestra, but it was a very exciting time. I was getting paid $45 a week, which seemed like a fortune to me. Equally important, I was accepted as a saxophone player by the other musicians in the orchestra, who went out of their way to help the young kid from Yonkers.

I played nightly with the orchestra at the Edison Hotel on Broadway. We also made two Shep Field records, which were nine saxophones and four rhythm instruments. Shep was evolving variations on a concept he developed called "Rippling Rhythm."

At the end of the two-week stint, Shep told me that I fit in so well that he wanted me to have a permanent spot with the band, including an opportunity to go on the road. "Mr. Field," I told him with a heavy heart, "there's nothing I'd like better, but we're going to war and I'm going to be drafted."

"What are you going to do in the meantime?" he asked me.

"Have as much fun as I can," I told him.

"Okay," he shrugged. "If you want to be a schmuck, be a schmuck."

I went back to Mrs. Fuchs's boarding house and was soon broke again, surviving off pickup jobs playing with little bands wherever I could. One day Frank Chase took out the most beautiful saxophone I had ever seen — a gold-plated Selma. "I just picked this up and you can have it for $115," he told me.

A gold-plated Selma for $115. There was a different kind of timbre, a different kind of sound that came out of a gold-plated Selma. I was in awe of that beautiful instrument. I took the subway to Yonkers and told my father about the Selma and how much it cost. It brought the saddest look to his eyes I could ever remember. "There's nothing I wouldn't give you if I could, but I can't come up with that kind of money." It was only $115 but might as well have been $100,000.

I went back to Frank and told him that I couldn't raise the money for the Selma. "Borrow it," he said. "On what?" I replied. It was the first time he realized how poor I really was. "I'll have to sell the Selma to someone else," he said. "But I think I have to get you some jobs."

He got me work with the Claude Thornhill and Charlie Spivak bands at the Glen Allen Casino. I had never seen their books, the collection of their music in written form that musicians generally had to study for a while before they were able to play with a group. But I was able to sight-read, and this allowed me to integrate quickly and easily. I was making a living as a musician, playing with other bands, including Art Mooney, on such gigs as the

Pick Ohio Hotel in Youngstown, Ohio, with its famous "all stainless steel dance floor." I even played briefly with the Benny Goodman orchestra. I also learned by watching other people perform. I was now making $55 a week, which was phenomenal money at the time.

But I was right when I told Shep Field that my days as a musician were numbered, and in September 1942 — right after the summer when I met Florence — I signed up with the United States Coast Guard. Abe had gone into the service the previous February. Although he was thirty-seven years old, the armed forces needed first-class cooks. He never went to boot camp. He got three stripes right away. He became part of the teams that ran the big kitchens and soon was feeding 15,000 men a day. Dave was exempted because he supported our parents.

I got my notice from Uncle Sam to report for duty in November. The night before I left I listened to the recording of Marcel Mule playing Jacques Ibert's *Concertino da Camera* before I went to bed. It was so gorgeous. I thought if I could play like that I would be the happiest person in the world.

At 4:00 a.m. I kissed my mother and father good-bye. I walked up to Main Street, thinking all along, like a lot of other guys did, that this might be the last time I'd ever see my parents.

I got on the trolley, which took me to Van Cortlandt Park in the Bronx. I then got the subway at 242nd Street and rode all the way down to Chambers Street.

I walked into the induction center and saw all these young men. We stripped for physicals, which was a strange sensation. Being examined naked with a couple of hundred other men around is not my cup of tea. When the physicals were over, we all raised our right hands and took our oath and we were in the service.

All of a sudden a guy yells out that everyone with the last names beginning with the letters A through L go to this side of the room, M through Z go to the other side of the room. Little did I know how lucky I was going to be. M through Z went to Parris Island, South Carolina, to be trained for combat. A through L were sent to Manhattan Beach in Brooklyn.

When you go through the gates and they close behind you, you are now the property of the United States Coast Guard. It was a funny feeling. I remember thinking, you can't go outside anymore without a pass or a voucher from an officer. That's it. The first night in the barracks, when it got quiet, there was a lot of whimpering going on. It was the first time away from home for many of us. A lot of guys were crying, including me.

I spent the next few months in boot training, which was tough, but no worse than the basic training everyone else had to go through in the military. I also went through additional training for captain of the port (COPT). We had to learn how to keep track of all the planes, jeeps, tires, weaponry, and other materials on the piers. In 1942 I got to spend the Christmas holiday liberty with Florence.

The day after Christmas I came back to Manhattan Beach and the announcement came, "All personnel whose last names begin with A to L pack your sea bags; you're being shipped out."

The base was shaped like an elongated L. We were marching down toward the corner. We knew that there would be trucks around that corner. If they were trailer trucks, we were going to be shipped someplace on land, somewhere in the continental United States. If there were troop trucks with benches, we were going to be shipped overseas.

As we turned the corner, there they

were. Troop trucks. You could hear the gasps and the "oh boys" from the crowd. We were going overseas. We were going into combat and there was a good chance we were going to get hurt or die.

Our platoon leader was named Whitey. He liked to kid around. "I hope you guys have your whites on top." Whites were the thin summer uniforms, which meant we were going on a ship. And this was December! The war was going strong in the South Pacific. We thought we were being shipped to Guadalcanal. I thought it was only a matter of time before we were there. It was the Coast Guard's job to bring in all of the troops, heavy machinery, and equipment and unload the barges under fire. I was picturing myself under a truck, being used to provide ballast to get a jeep out of the sand.

"You guys are going to G'watus Canal," Whitey mumbled. My buddies and I were all looking at each other in disgust. "How do you like that for luck," we muttered. Whitey smiled. We couldn't figure out why he was smiling. Was he that sadistic?

"Don't you guys get it? You're going to Gowanus Canal. Pier 1, Brooklyn!" They were sending us to Brooklyn! You never saw so many cookies, cakes, and salamis coming out of bags. The celebration on the truck was enormous. We went from despair to euphoria in a heartbeat.

Not only were we going to be in the country, we were going to be in New York, which meant that I could be near Florence. I was part of a group that became affectionately known as the "Subway Commandos."

It turned out a lot of equipment was being shipped overseas though the Port of New York that needed to be guarded and counted every night and every morning to make sure nothing was stolen. The concern was not only pilfering. We also had to make sure that none of the volatile equipment, including the 105- and 155-millimeter shells and the 75-millimeter tank shells, as well as 500- and 1,000-pound bombs, blew up.

On the docks, we were each given a pistol before each watch, which we had to turn in at the end of the shift. We were given sixteen bullets, six for the pistol and ten for the belt. All bullets had to be accounted for at the end of the watch, too.

It was a job you had to do. In winter on the wooden planked Brooklyn docks, the cold rose up from the water and it was brutal. You wore the entire contents of your duffel bag on watch — your peacoat, two pairs of long underwear, three pairs of socks, all of your T-shirts, and a watch cap. And if your mother gave you a sweater, you put that on, too. It was tough, monotonous, and very, very cold.

The shifts were six hours long: from 7:00 a.m. to 1:00 p.m., 1:00 p.m. to 7:00 p.m., 7:00 p.m. to 1:00 a.m., and 1:00 a.m. till 7:00 a.m.

When watch ended at one o'clock in the morning, we often got sandwiches from Father Duffy's. Father Duffy's was an organization that provided coffee and sandwiches to soldiers when the military kitchen wasn't open.

One night, all of a sudden, we heard sirens. I thought we were being invaded. We were told to report to the ammo shack, where each of us was issued a .45-caliber submachine gun. It was called a rising machine gun because as you fired it, the barrel rose. We were instructed to put one arm on top of the barrel to keep it down; that was all the training we received in the use of that particular weapon. I concluded that the rising machine gun was made by Woolworth's.

We were all put onto huge lifeboats with motors and took off out of the canal into the harbor, all the way to a railroad pier in Hoboken, New Jersey. I remember watching some of the guys in the boat scratching their heads with the muzzles of their weapons. They didn't inspire a lot of confidence. "Fellas, these are machine guns!" I remember telling them.

The Coast Guard was the first group in. Behind us was a battalion of marines (800 men) and an army brigade. Ten square blocks were sealed off.

I was ordered to go up into the wheelhouse on the ferry to keep watch. I could see everything coming up and down the river. There were planes and destroyers everywhere. We didn't know what was going on. The order came down: "If you see anything move in the water near the dock, open fire."

At about four in the morning, one guy opened fire at the dock. Then 250 men with machine guns started shooting, all firing at the same spot. I remember dropping to the floor of the wheelhouse. The shooting went on for five minutes. I was afraid to move.

As dawn broke, I saw that the better part of the pier next to us had been shot up. It had been a false alarm. The soldier who started the shooting had shot at a piece of wood that was floating in the water. I still had the view of the entire river from the wheelhouse. At about 7:00 a.m., from nowhere a day liner started heading toward us and a railroad train started to back up to the pier. The boat docked and the lines were secured. A company of British marines started to get off. Each of them was a big bruiser with a rifle and a fixed bayonet.

British marines, I thought. What were they doing here? Are we at war with England? The marines formed a double line from the gangplank of the ship to the train. A train car was backed up, and I saw a man wearing a derby hat and smoking a huge cigar walk off the gangplank through the paired marines. "Holy smoke," I thought. "It's Winston Churchill! He's going to Hyde Park to see Roosevelt!"

Seeing Churchill was exciting, but otherwise life in the Coast Guard was routine, happily so, and monotonous. For each six-hour shift you got twelve hours off. And after every fourth shift you got twenty-four hours off. You never got to sleep at the same time for more than five days in a row, which after a few months made you a little disoriented. Morale was very low. The guys didn't care if they were put on report. They didn't change their sheets. Some guys would actually try to shoot their big toe off. If you hit your target, you either got discharged or you were punished. After you got out of the infirmary, you got sent to the brig and questioned by a psychiatrist.

While I was stationed in the Brooklyn barracks, I met a man named Vernon Duke. He was an accomplished composer who wrote the classic songs "Autumn in New York," "April in Paris," "Taking a Chance on Love," and "I Can't Get Started," which became Bunny Berrigan's theme song. He wrote the score for *Cabin in the Sky* as well as classical music. Vernon's real name was Vladimir Alexander Dukelsky. He was a Russian who had immigrated to the United States with his family in 1921, and at forty years of age he enlisted in the service out of a love for the United States and for what it had done for him.

Vernon held the rank of coxswain (the equivalent of sergeant). Vernon was very nearsighted and was too proud to wear his glasses. He couldn't do close order drill. He couldn't tell his left oblique from his right. Our friendship began when I told him to hang on to the collar of my uniform to help him march in the same direction as the rest of the men. I asked him once how he passed the physical. "I was so patriotic that I tried every branch of the service. I insisted on serving somewhere," he said. "They finally figured I could do the least amount of damage in the Coast Guard," he joked.

The officers on the base knew Vernon as a famous Broadway composer. To me, he was just a guy that needed my help. I had no idea who he was outside the service. But I soon learned.

I was looking for a reason to get off the piers. Being there was driving me crazy, but I was looking for a more constructive solution than shooting off my big toe. Vernon gave me the idea to start a band. I went around to the barracks and started canvassing the men looking for musicians. I found nine saxophone players, one guitar player, and one bass player. Not one trumpet player or anyone who could play the piano, other than Vernon.

I went to Lieutenant Tom Silverman, who was the base commander. I said, "Lieutenant, sir, you know what would be a smart move? An orchestra. Morale is horrible. The guys are shooting their toes off to get out of duty. Most of the guys don't care if you throw them in the brig. They're as comfortable there as they are on the outside. In fact, in the brig, they don't have to go on watch and freeze to death.

"I'd like to get an orchestra down here. We should build a recreation hall. There's no place for the guys to even sit down and smoke a cigarette, and no PX. We could start an orchestra and put up a stage and get girls. If we had dances here, morale would skyrocket."

"Where are we going to get the building?" he asked.

"We can build a place to dance out of the barracks," I told him. "We could get a spotlight and use denim to make a curtain and have a real show."

"Where are you going to get the girls?" he asked.

Where do we get the girls?

I was just an apprentice seaman with one little white stripe telling a two bar lieutenant where to get girls. Didn't he know there was a war on? "There is a shortage of able-bodied men," I told him. There were no young guys hanging out on the corners. We knew exactly where to send the trucks to get the girls, like the USO. "If the girls of New York City heard there was a dance and they were going to be escorted and guarded by four SPs (Shore Patrol), they would feel safe."

The lieutenant thought about my idea for a few moments and agreed. With the help of a bull gang (the group that built whatever you needed), we put up a recreation hall the size of four barracks with a stage from the ground up. I dug the ditches for the plumbing, and I was also handing the stacked walls down to the other men to build the floor. It was the military version of Judy Garland and Mickey Rooney putting on a show. We even trucked in female dancers.

We instituted a rule that no girl could go out for a cigarette with a man. They had to go alone. We put out an announcement: "Any sailor caught outside the recreation hall with a girl will get a full court martial." We really wanted the recreation hall to work.

I went to see Shep Field in Manhattan and asked for some of his arrangements to copy. "Anything for the service," he said. He not only gave me the arrangements but also had them broken down and copied at no charge. Then he gave me cab fare to get back to the base. I realized how really generous some people were to servicemen during the war.

Finally Friday night came, and we had music and dancing, coffee and sandwiches, and most importantly young women. All of our hard work paid off. Everyone shaped up. All of a sudden morale improved and so did performance and attitude. None of these guys wanted to wind up in the brig on a Friday night and miss the dance and the girls. If you got just two demerits, you weren't allowed to go to the dance. You never saw such snapping to, saluting, and "yes-sirring" in the history of the armed forces. Not one sailor was on report. I learned another very valuable lesson: Women are a very powerful influence on men.

The PX sold more Brylcreem, Skin Bracer, and shaving cream than ever before. They ran out of soap, perfumes, aftershave, and anything else that smelled good. The laundry was never so busy. Even the barracks smelled great. The dance was a big success. Between the musical numbers, I entertained the men. I did the wartime and peacetime airplane movie routines that Dave and I had written, which the men loved.

Vernon Duke and I became very close friends and he worked on arrangements for the revues. We got a guy from the band named Bert Kempe to help with the arrangements. Vernon played piano with the group of saxophonists. We were so popular we were asked to play at dances on other bases. We also got to play at the USO club on Broadway. That was the big time.

With the success of the weekly dances, I thought that since we have the band, the hall, and the seats, why not do a revue about life on the piers. So with the experiences I had in sketch comedy from the Catskills, I started to write a show, which I called "Six On, Twelve Off," basing it on the base watch shifts. I did sketches about different officers and about guys and their different habits, what happens when the cold air hits them on patrol at the docks. The officers were so enthusiastic about the show that they loaned us their jackets to use as costumes, which we had to return the next day, cleaned and pressed. We did sketches about the cooks and the drivers. We didn't miss anyone. We even made fun of the commanding officer.

We opened the show on a Friday night and were a big hit. The guys wanted to see it again. The guys who were on watch also wanted to see it. The brass loved the show too; even the admiral came up to see it. They decided that the show should be sent around the Third Naval District to entertain the soldiers on all the piers. The men loved to see a show that was based on what they did. People enjoy what they know about.

Whenever Bob Hope would perform at a

base, the first thing he would ask when he landed was, "What's the name of the son of a bitch who runs this place?" And he would work the names of the commanding officers, key personnel, and a little local dirt into the show. We did the same thing, changing the routines for each base. It was great.

I did songs and impressions, building my repertoire. I didn't have a full act yet. I had the airplane routine that I had developed with Dave. Mostly I did pieces of business, including an impression of Hitler talking to Donald Duck and a gangster talking on the telephone. "I'm sorry," he says as he is getting machine-gunned, "I gotta hang up now. I can't hear what you're saying. There's just too many bullets." I wrote songs with a lieutenant commander who was the chief medical officer of the base. I would argue with him over the songs. He would genially admonish me: "You're saying no, no, no to a lieutenant commander?" It was all great fun.

But I also had other things on my mind. During this time, Florence and I went to the wedding of one of her girlfriends. I remember looking at her and fumbling for words.

"Do you think, should we?" I said.

"Do you want to marry me?" she asked.

"Yes. That's what I wanted to say."

Florence, as she has done for sixty years since, helped me find the words.

In one of the smartest moves I ever made in my life, actually *the* smartest move, I married Florence on July 17, 1943. Dave threw the wedding for us at the Moskowitz & Lupowitz restaurant on the Lower East Side in Manhattan. It was a small ceremony with just the immediate families.

Coxswain Vernon Duke was my best man, though he was about to become an ex-coxswain. He and the Coast Guard had decided that for the good of the service, it would be best for them to part ways. He was going back to the civilian theater to write another musical comedy. After the ceremony, Vernon played piano and I played the saxophone for the guests.

I couldn't get a forty-eight-hour pass for my honeymoon, but I did manage two twenty-four-hour passes. I had to wake up at five o'clock in the morning, leave our room at the Hotel Manhattan, and go back to the base in the middle of my honeymoon, check in, and then go back to the hotel.

By the time you read this, Florence Levy Caesar and I will have been married for sixty years. By the time you finish this book, you will understand that the reason I am alive today to tell my story is because of Florence. She has stood by me through the tests of time and great adversity. She provided emotional support for me and our family, saved my life countless times, and always loved me. She is the most beautiful version of the Rock of Gibraltar I will ever see in my life.

Florence married me before I became a star. She got on the roller coaster with me at the very beginning. People would always tell me that Florence deserved a chest full of medals for putting up with me. So I actually went out and found a chest full of medals at a pawnshop and gave them to her. After sixty years of marriage, there isn't a day that I don't wake up with a sense of gratitude and love for the woman who has been my best friend and partner, the person who kept me alive when by all accounts I should have been long gone. When Max Liebman later told her, "Your husband is going to be a big, big star," she prophetically and protectively said, "Couldn't he just be a little star?"

Marriages in general don't last as long as ours. The odds are even worse for marriages between people in show business. Even the ones that last as long don't match our level of passion and chemistry.

Florence didn't marry me for money or fame. At the time I had neither. When we got married, I was making $66 a month. I didn't have the money to buy her anything. I was the Sidney that wrote her love letters and cute little songs that I would sing to her, like this one:

I wrote you a song for your birthday,
I wrote it 'cause I want you to know,
That I couldn't buy anything real
To show you darling just how I feel.
So I wrote you a song for your birthday,
I wrote it 'cause I want you to know,
That I still remember the third of September
Means happy birthday, dear Florence, to you.

Am I still smitten? You bet.

Chapter 4

TARS AND SPARS

Vernon Duke and I stayed friends even after he was discharged from the Coast Guard. He was a good man. Every time I had liberty and left the base to spend time with Florence, he would invite me to his apartment on Lexington Avenue and East 35th Street in Manhattan for a decent meal. "You should never see Florence on an empty stomach," he would say. He was worried that I'd blow my entire monthly allotment on the first restaurant Florence and I came to.

I so enjoyed the time I spent with Florence. Things were great between us. But I began to hate hotel rooms and couldn't wait for the war to be over, so we could live together as man and wife.

Vernon also invited me to his Broadway production of *Cabin in the Sky*. He took me backstage and introduced me to the actors. "Dis man is very talented in many vays," he would say, pointing to me. "He plays the clarinet and the saxophone, he can sing, and he can also make people laugh."

One day I tried to contact Vernon, but he had moved out of his apartment and left no forwarding address, no note. Within a week, though, Lieutenant Silverman called me in. He was puzzled. "I've seen orders for one person, an admiral, a captain. But below the rank of captain, deployment orders usually came in for thousands of men. I've never seen an order from Washington for just one seaman in my entire career." But he was holding a set of orders that one Seaman First Class Sidney Caesar, serial number 646717, report to the Coast Guard barracks, Biltmore Hotel, Palm Beach, Florida. He didn't understand that.

With barely enough time to say good-bye to Florence, I boarded the train bound for Florida. I realized that I had never been farther south than Asbury Park. I didn't know why I had been summoned to Florida until I reached the lobby of the fancy Biltmore Hotel, which had been converted to a Coast Guard station. A very familiar face greeted me. It was Vernon Duke. He was wearing a Coast Guard officer's uniform of full lieutenant.

I was both stunned and happy to see him. I was also confused. "Why are you in uniform?" I asked. "You're a civilian."

"Not any more," he said.

The army produced its own show for the troops and so did the air force. The navy said, "We don't do that. Let the Coast Guard do the show." So the Coast Guard put Vernon together with Howard Dietz, a great Broadway producer and lyricist, to write the show, which they were calling *Tars and Spars*. Vernon had requested my presence for the cast, which was granted. That explained the order for just one seaman.

I went from the cold and dismal Brooklyn port to balmy and swanky Palm Beach. One day I was fixing toilets in Brooklyn, the next I was rehearsing with a big movie star like Victor Mature and a choreographer like Gower Champion. It was a charm. I knew in my bones that the show would be a hit.

It was also there that Vernon introduced me to Max Liebman, the civilian director of the show. People who worked in the Catskills knew Max as an impresario who was affectionately called the "Ziegfeld of the borscht belt." He was a showman who was born in Vienna. When he came to this country he spent years writing and producing vaudeville acts, and he'd worked at everything from Catskill tummler to Broadway producer.

Max Liebman was a great collector of talent. In Camp Tamiment, which was an adult summer camp in the Pocono Mountains, he wrote, produced, and directed original revues for the fifteen hundred guests. One of Max's Tamiment shows, *The Straw Hat Revue*, even made it to Broadway. It was also at Tamiment that he discovered Danny Kaye and met and worked with Sylvia Fine, another writer/performer and the future Mrs. Kaye.

Max helped Danny develop his act and went to Hollywood with him and Sylvia. He worked on Danny's first film, *Up in Arms*, in 1940 and then became a staff writer at MGM. I knew he was a man to pay attention to. He was a short man, smoked cigars, and had, I later learned, a collection of very bad toupees.

I did the airplane sketch for Max, and he worked with me to retool it into a big theatrical piece. It became "Wings over Bombinschissel." He took out the peacetime component and had me focus on the wartime part of the sketch. "We're going to do an out-and-out parody of *Wings*," he said. "There will be an American ace that is always smiling and a German ace that is always snarling. We'll have them in typical Hollywood World War I dogfights, with the smiling American winning." He helped turn Dave's and my idea into a nine-minute routine.

I did all the sound effects with my mouth, including the starting of the airplane engines and the throttle. The sketch was based on the premise that German airplanes sounded very irritating, while American planes had a wholesome sound and looked clean-cut and were always smiling. "It was always raining," I began. "Never a clear day . . . there are two smiling men, one with a mustache and one without a mustache. That's for girls that like men with mustaches and for those that don't like men with mustaches." There was a romance in the piece, with the two pilots fighting over the girl: "I'll take the plane up, you marry Jane. No, I'll take the plane up and you marry Jane." I knock out my pal and get into the plane. "I told you to marry Jane!"

Although I was the only performer, I began to people the stage with characters and imaginary props. Max liked what I could do, and he and Vernon kept adding to my part on the show. I would play the saxophone and I also did my conversation between Hitler and Donald Duck in double-talk.

Max also helped me develop a few more routines. When Max left the show he said to me, "After the war, I want you to come see me." "If I survive the war," I replied, "I certainly will."

The revue toured nationally for almost a year. The proceeds went to the Coast Guard relief fund. It was billed as *"Tars and Spars,* with Victor Mature, Gower Champion, and Fifty Others." The fifty others was forty-nine plus me.

During our run in Philadelphia, the commandant of the Coast Guard (the equivalent of a general with four stars), Russell R. Waesche, came down to see the show. He liked my performance. Captain Ellis Reed-Hill was the admiral's aide-de-camp, and he brought the commandant to meet me after the show and shake my hand. "Caesar," he said, "you're a great addition to the show. Well done."

I was always an anxious performer. During the course of our run, Captain Reed-Hill noticed that I had begun throwing up every day, so he arranged for a special dispensation from the Coast Guard, which enabled Florence to travel with me throughout the rest of the tour. With Florence with me I was much less nervous and was able to focus on performing. I can never thank Captain (later Admiral) Reed-Hill enough for being so helpful and instrumental in my career. He was my guardian angel.

We started to hear scuttlebutt that Columbia Pictures had bought the rights to the show. I could barely contain my enthusiasm: I was going to be in a movie. But when we got to Hollywood to do the film version of *Tars and Spars*, there was a strike on. We couldn't shoot the film, but we were all reporting to the studio every day anyhow. I was getting a $10 per diem from the studio. Seventy dollars a week in 1944! That in addition to the $66 a month from the Coast Guard. I felt very rich.

The first movie set I ever visited was *A Thousand and One Nights* with Cornell Wilde. To see a real Hollywood set with costumes and Evelyn Keyes was amazing. I watched a scene being filmed where a rider was being shot with an arrow while speeding by on horseback. The rider was shot with a real arrow that got him smack in the chest. He had a cork vest under his robes backed up by a solid piece of steel that caught the arrow. The archer never missed. I had never seen a stuntman work before. He took the risk of a real arrow.

Florence and I lived on Taft Avenue in a

one-room cold water flat with a hot plate. I had a car now, a 1928 Ford, for which I paid $190.

The movie plot for *Tars and Spars* was simple and typical of the armed forces romance movies of the time. Alfred Drake (who replaced Victor Mature in the film) played a Coast Guardsman who has been on shore duty for three years despite his efforts to be sent into action. His nearest approach to sea duty was being on a harbor-moored life raft for twenty-one days as part of an experiment with a new type of vitamin gum for the government. He meets a SPAR, the equivalent of a WAC (played by Janet Blair), who was sent to take over his communications job. By things he leaves unsaid, she thinks his life raft experience was the result of a ship-wreck at sea. A love story was added to the mix. I played the friend of the leading man, Alfred Drake's pal, Chuck Enders, appropriately nicknamed "Yonkers." In those days, the comic was always the leading man's best friend. Phil Silvers used to be cast in that role. I also had a love interest, Penny, played by Jeff Donnell. A young Hugh Beaumont, who was most famous for later playing the father in *Leave It to Beaver*, was also in the movie.

I was the voice of every sad-sack service-man, hanging around with my buddies, rehearsing what I would say to my superior if I ever got the nerve up: "Now look, chief. Either you take me in to see the captain or I'll pluck the braid off your sleeve and ram it down your throat. Who do you think you are, a human being? How's that sound, Howie?"

If the Catskills were college, Hollywood was graduate school for me as an entertainer. The strike lasted for nine months, which sidelined production, but it gave me the opportunity to talk to many different people and watch and learn. I was getting an education in dancing, musical direction, and movie staging. I would spend hours listening to the music that the great orchestra of the brilliant and prolific Columbia Pictures musical director Morris Stoloff put together. I would watch him score other movies as well, and listen to him talk about the importance of music in a movie.

At Columbia I got to meet and work with a talented dancer and choreographer named Jack Cole. His assistant was a young woman named Gwen Verdon, who was also the captain of the chorus. Jack Cole was an original. He started the new wave of dancing that Bob Fosse took to the next level, which included knee slides and other great innovative moves. Bob Fosse was in one of the shows that Jack choreographed and watched him like a hawk. Jack was a real genius, but he was crazy. He would choreograph numbers around you. During one of the breaks, we had time to kill, so Jack started ordering props, including a horse's bridle, ears, tail, saddle, and a mane, and improvised an entire dance routine. He looked like a da Vinci horse. And he did it all for his own amusement and to entertain the friends around him.

Jack Cole was a solo dancer and a choreographer, but Hollywood didn't know exactly what to do with him. I would watch him off camera in awe. There wasn't a physical angle he couldn't reach. His movements were like silk. Although I was never formally trained as a dancer, I had a natural sense of rhythm and always kept in shape via a daily regimen of exercises, including push-ups and sit-ups. Jack showed me great moves, which I was able to assimilate and execute.

I had to do a number called "I Love Eggs." While on the mess line to get food, I was distracted by server Penny, who was pursuing me relentlessly. She piled a lot of eggs on my tray and I kept holding my plate there. I was oblivious to the big sign overhead — TAKE ALL YOU WANT, BUT EAT ALL YOU TAKE.

I see the sign and get nervous: "Oh boy . . . if the chief sees me with all these eggs on the platter." And the chief comes over to me and says "You like eggs that much?" I respond, "Do I love eggs!" and launch into a big number:

More than the pirate loves the shekel
More than the brewer loves his keg
More than a barefoot boy loves his cycle
More than a chambermaid could love
*   the porter*
I love eggs!

I was dancing on the tables and flying all over the room. Jack had me doing things that I never thought I could do. Jumping onto the table, I launched into different double-talk languages: I did a Mexican hat dance, I played a German cook, dancing to the tunes of "Three Blind Mice" and the *William Tell Overture.*

Another song I did in the movie was called "He's a Hero," which involved marching and dancing. The technicians on the film slowed the footage down and transcribed the words for me so that it could be reedited and the vocals would be clearer. These guys liked me and believed in me. I learned one of my most valuable lessons: How important the technical crew is to the success of a performer. They can make you or break you.

One of the last scenes to be filmed for the picture was my airplane-movie number. Initially, it wasn't supposed to be in the movie. The director, Alfred Green, who would later direct *The Jolson Story* with Larry Parks, had never seen me do the piece. He asked how long would it take to do the number, I told him, "eight and a half minutes." He then asked, "How long will it take to shoot the scene?" I said, "As long as it will take me to do it." I had fine-tuned the routine to the point where I could do it in one take — eight and a half minutes flat. I told him how to do his long and medium shots, his close-ups and his reaction shots. We shot the entire scene in one morning.

The head of Columbia Studios, the legendary Harry Cohn, didn't know about the airplane number in advance. When he found out, he said, "Eight and a half minutes for only one person! You can show four world wars and eight love stories in eight and a half minutes!" "Let's see what the audience thinks," Alfred Drake said.

When the movie was screened for the test audiences in Santa Barbara, all of the response cards that were filled out at the end of the movie said, "Who's the blond kid that did the airplane number?" The cards were all dumped on Cohn's desk. He finally sat down and watched the scene. He yelled (his regular form of communication): "I got talent right in front of me and no one tells me! The scene stays in the picture!"

As shooting was wrapping up on *Tars and Spars*, I was approached by Lieutenant Commander Milton Bren, who was our Coast Guard liaison to Columbia Pictures. Milton was involved in real estate in civilian life, but had a lot of contacts in the movie business. He introduced me to the songwriters Sammy Cahn and Jule Styne. Offering me $500 a week to manage me, Milton said he would make deals with the movie studios for my services, the way big producers like David O. Selznick did in those days. I signed with him.

Milton gave me a thousand dollar signing bonus. I took the check to the bank and got a thousand one dollar bills. I went back to our apartment and surprised Florence. I threw the money in the air, and it came down like confetti on the bed. "That's the first thousand," I said. And then the money went right back to the bank.

The studio sent Florence and me to New York to do publicity for *Tars and Spars*. Milton Bren got me a Beverly Hills tailor, Jack Taylor, whom I have been buying clothes from ever since. The studio put us up at the Pierre Hotel on Fifth Avenue. It was a large suite with its own grand piano. I had never seen anything that opulent before. It was like being on a movie set.

While I was in New York, I learned that my father was very ill. He had cancer, which was something no one talked about in those days. I didn't take the news well. Florence kept me from falling apart.

I picked up the phone and called Al Rylander, who turned out to be one of the best friends I ever had. He was the publicity director for Columbia Pictures in New York. I told him about how ill my father was and that I wanted him to see a preview of *Tars and Spars*. Al switched one of the previews from the Loews Delancey downtown to the Loews Paradise in the Bronx, which was much closer to Yonkers.

We went to Yonkers on the night of the preview and drove my father to the theater. He was in his seventies, frail, and a shell of his former powerful self. He watched the movie and I watched him, never taking my eyes off him.

He said nothing during the film, and for the entire ride home. When he sat down in his living room, he spoke.

"Sidney, you say you make $500 a week."

"Yes, Papa," I said.

"That's a lot of money. Put some away," he said. "If you take care, you'll be all right." It was his way of expressing approval and happiness at what he had just seen.

He passed away a few months later and I flew back from California for his funeral. The studio paid for a first-class airplane ticket. Dave told me that my father had seen the reviews of *Tars and Spars*. The movie had opened to less than glowing notices and did not do particularly well at the box office. Fortunately, I got very good reviews. Wanda Hale in the New York *Daily News* wrote: "Sid Caesar is a real comedy find. His interpretation of an Air Force movie is alone worth the price of admission."

I did a second movie while I was in Hollywood, which Milton Bren set up for me, called *The Guilt of Janet Ames*, with Melvyn Douglas and Rosalind Russell. They wanted me to do a standup routine. I wrote a piece with Robert Allen, who was a songwriter with a great sense of humor on staff at Columbia Pictures.

After the war, I was discharged from the service. Florence and I stayed in California for a while, in the hopes of my developing a movie career. Dave flew out a few times to see us. He was now working at the post office. It was a big deal at the time for him to come to California. A round-trip ticket was $300. It was also a ten-hour flight. But Dave wasn't going to let a significant amount of time go by without seeing me and making sure I was okay. He would get off the plane with a big smile, armed with stories he spontaneously made up about every subject. Once Dave stayed with us for two months. He, Florence, and I never laughed so hard.

Mel Brooks has made no secret of the fact that the inspiration for the scene in *Blazing Saddles* where a character punches a horse and knocks it down really happened in my life while I was living in California. Florence and I were horseback riding in Griffith Park. When our horses reached a stream, Florence's horse just lay down in it and started to roll over. Had the horse rolled over any further, Florence would have been crushed. I was terrified.

I jumped off my horse and told Florence to jump away. But she didn't move. So I grabbed the horse and got it to get up. And then I hit the horse. I was just so mad. I didn't hurt the horse, and I didn't knock him down like the character did in *Blazing Saddles*, but I was so furious that the horse would put my wife in a dangerous situation. To hit an animal is nuts. It's crazy. But I did it. I am a great lover of animals. But when my wife's safety is involved, everything goes by the boards. It happened in a flash. I never deliberately hurt an animal in my life. Mel, on the other hand, was a different story.

Some scripts came my way. I was offered the lead in *The Jolson Story*, but I knew from the start that I wasn't an impersonator, so I passed on the role. I was always offered the part of the star's best friend. Every leading man had a pal, a sidekick, who was a comedian.

I didn't want to be the best friend; I wanted to be the leading man. My timing in Hollywood was off. The era of the great comedians had ended a decade earlier. The days of Chaplin, Keaton, and W. C. Fields were over, and it was years before Hollywood would let a comedian play the legitimate lead in a movie.

A lot of life is about timing — being born at the right time. When World War II started, I was a doorman at the Capitol Theatre. And when the war ended, I was a comedic performer in Hollywood. But as good as that was, I got very few parts. I would get up in the morning, play tennis, and go swimming. A telephone call would upset my routine. But I was raised to be a worker, and I needed to work.

Tony Martin was the first guy I worked with after I got out of the service. It was at the Chicago Theater, and Tony not only put my name up in lights under his but even in the same size. I walked outside the theater with Florence and just stared at my name in lights, musing with Florence about how far I had come. I never forgot Tony Martin's magnanimous gesture.

One day in 1946 I received a visit from a man named Monte Proser, who staged shows at the Copacabana nightclub in New York. We had met at a party in Hollywood, and he had told me how much he liked my work in *Tars and Spars*. "How would you like to do a couple of months at the Copa?" he asked.

"I have no material," I told him.

"You'll get something," he said.

I called the only person I knew who could give me the right advice, Max Liebman. "You're not being used right in

Hollywood," he told me. "I will personally help you write an act for the Copa."

I ended my contractual relationship with Milton Bren. Florence and I packed our clothes and pots and pans and moved back to New York, where Max and I sat down to write. We added three other numbers to the nine-minute airplane sketch, and I had a half hour act, which was all the time you got at the Copa back then. They wanted turnover. We did three shows a night: 8:00 p.m., 11:00 p.m., and 2:30 in the morning. I was on the bill with a singer and the Copa Girls chorus line.

I opened at the Copa on New Year's Day, 1947. I followed an engagement of the legendary comedian Joe E. Louis. I was the sacrificial lamb. No one wanted to follow Joe E. Louis, especially on New Year's Day. Guys had worked for years to get to the Copa, and it was the first night-club I ever played. I didn't know how I would do. I didn't know whether anyone knew me. The place was jammed with people. And I was plenty scared.

Much to my surprise, as soon as I started, there were great laughs. The next day, the newspapers reported that I was a hit. I was amazed and pleased.

After the two-month engagement was

over, Max introduced me to his agent at William Morris. "They'll get you bookings all over the country. I'll go with you. You've got a lot to learn. We want you to be ready for a lot of things that could happen to us in the future."

Max was planning a future for us. He was speaking "we" and "us." I had found yet another protector and mentor in my life.

Chapter 5

A SHOW OR A STEAK

With Max Liebman alongside me and my brother Dave meeting us in certain cities, I did a tour of the nightclub circuit. Traveling all over the country, I was perfecting my act as a "single." In the beginning, I was very inexperienced; I literally "didn't know stage right from stage left." Max wasn't a teacher per se, but I still had the opportunity to learn. For his part, Max was intent on not making any mistakes with me. He was going to nurture me and ride with me to the top. But Max didn't expect me to learn and to grow as rapidly and as successfully as I did.

Danny Kaye was the big star at the time, and he set the standard for film and musical comedy. He was Max's first protégé. Max had written Danny's early routines with Sylvia Fine and was used to writing in that same vein. I told Max I didn't want to imitate Danny Kaye. I wanted to develop my own style off what I had learned from Chaplin,

Keaton, Fields, and Laurel and Hardy.

I also met Martha Raye around this time. She was playing at the old Cairo Club in Washington, D.C., and I was playing the nearby Rumanian. She was not only one of the best comediennes I had ever heard, she also had one of the greatest jazz voices I ever heard, outside of Ella Fitzgerald and Sarah Vaughan. I had finished my set, and Dave and I went to see her at a late show. I just sat there and listened to her sing till the end of the show at 2:30 in the morning. She kept the piano player and then continued to sing for a small group of us until 4:00 a.m. It was a rare and unforgettable moment in my life.

Dave and I were going to visit a cousin the next night. "I'll come with you," she said. Our cousin, the mild-mannered optometrist, never expected to see Martha Raye! They never really captured Martha properly in movies. They only knew from classic beauty. Martha always made herself less attractive because she played the clown.

The first night I appeared at the Club Charles in Baltimore, there wasn't one laugh. Just little rumblings. After the show, I went to the owner and told him, "Look, you don't have to pay me. I'll just go home and we'll call it even." "Are you kidding?" he replied. "This is the quietest this place has been for any act. They've never paid attention. You're staying!" I was a silent hit. The next night the audience laughed. They caught on to what I was doing.

It was in Baltimore that I first met and befriended Zero Mostel. We had known each other by name and reputation. He was at the Chanticleer when I was at the Club Charles down the street. His show always ended later than mine did. I would catch the last half hour of his last set, and then we would go out and grab a bite to eat.

Zero was a gifted performer who will always be remembered for bringing Tevye to life in *Fiddler on the Roof* on Broadway. He was the one who came up with the business of softly snapping his fingers in the air as he looked up to God and sang. He put the "deedle deedle" in "If I Were a Rich Man." He would go off the script a lot, in *Fiddler* and in *The Producers*, much to the initial chagrin of writers and directors, but to the later pleasure of everyone, especially the audience.

On the nightclub stage, Zero was electric. He would imitate a piece of bacon frying and coffee percolating. He had boundless energy and could do anything.

One night there was a drunk sitting at a table at the foot of the stage. He began to heckle Zero. The heckler kept yelling, "Get off the stage, fatso! And fast!" Without missing a beat, Zero said, "And now my impression of a motorcycle!"

Zero started making the revving noises: "Vroom, vroom, vroom!" He moved to the back of the stage and then lunged upstage, jumped up, and landed on the heckler's table. "Is that fast enough for you?" he yelled, breaking the table. He scared the hell out of the whole place and probably ruined the guy's suit. He calmly walked over to me and we left the club to get something to eat. I was hysterical.

Zero was a wonderful man, but it was smart not to get him mad. He was also very extreme in his political views. He was in the "book," along with a lot of great writers like Dalton Trumbo and Ring Lardner Jr., who got blacklisted, and whose careers were crushed by Joe McCarthy. McCarthy would hold up toilet paper and babble, sounding like a poor imitation of Ed Sullivan. They had actually come after Lucille Ball and me, but they couldn't find anything on either of us. McCarthy's self-motivated crusade set the arts and democracy back many years.

Zero wasn't the only one it wasn't smart to get mad. In my youth, I was possessed with Herculean strength, and I had a temper, too. I could walk through walls without opening a door. I never instigated anything and never acted unprovoked. But there were moments . . .

Right after the war, it was still hard to buy a new car. I'd just gotten a 1941 Cadillac in good condition. It had 30,000 miles on it. I had it redone. I painted it and fixed it up inside, and put on new whitewall tires. It was my pride and joy. Dave and I went to Greenwich Village to see Zero perform. When we got to the Village, I parked near a fire hydrant, but just far enough to be sure that I wouldn't get a ticket. I left myself a little room in the back so that I could get out. I didn't want anyone touching my car. We were already crossing the street when we watched this guy pull up and use his car to push mine back so that he could get away from the fireplug. Then he squeezed into the space between my car and the fireplug.

There were two couples in the car — one in the front, one in the back. I walked over to the driver's window and said, "Look, I just had the car painted, and you're pushing my car. Would you please stop." His cold response was, "Take a walk." I was still calm. "I'm gonna ask you once more. You hit my car; I just had it painted. You can't get enough room." The response was still, "Take a walk."

I then said, "Do you remember being born?" He said he didn't understand the question. I said, "Do you remember what it felt like to come out of the womb?" He still didn't understand the question. I said, "Let me show you." I reached into the car and grabbed him by his lapels — one hand through the little window and one hand around, and began to pull. I nearly pulled him through the window. The guy was holding on to the steering wheel, but to no avail — his clothes started to rip. "Sid, let him go," Dave yelled. Dave was always the voice of reason. The man drove away.

Tars and Spars had raised my profile and made me a hot commodity on the East Coast. I got work right away. In addition to the Copacabana and the Latin Quarter, I was booked at the Roxy Theater in Manhattan's Rockefeller Center four times in one year. They loved me because I was different. I didn't tell jokes. There were 5,000 seats in the Roxy, and I used to open with my old friend the airplane number.

Don Appel, another old friend from the Catskills, had reintroduced me to Mel Brooks when I played the Copa. When I was at the Roxy he came by on his own and would hang around during the downtime. He also became friendly with my brothers, Abe and Dave, who spent a lot of time with me at the theater.

Max Liebman came to me one day and told me about a new revue opening on Broadway called *Make Mine Manhattan* that wanted me. Joe Hyman, a former sweater manufacturer with a year-round blinding tan, was the producer of the show and the money man. He came backstage after one of my performances. "I saw you with the airplane number," he began. He was already angling for a deal. He said, "Tell you what I'll do with you — I'll give you $250 a week."

I looked at him like he was crazy. I was already making $3,500 a week at the Roxy. The Copacabana was offering me $3,500 a week. This guy was offering me $250? To my shock, Max calmly said, "Take it. It's the best thing for you. You're going into a Broadway show, a whole new audience will see you, and it's a good step." I took the deal, but only on the condition that I got a two-week option: Joe Hyman and I could each terminate the arrangement with two weeks' notice.

The revue consisted of a series of sketches and songs, all about the island of Manhattan. Hyman had already signed up some top talent, including Davey Burns, one of the biggest comedians in the country. The cast also included Sheila Bond, Kyle MacDonnell, Biff McGuire, Julie Oshins, Joshua Shelley, and Max Showalter. One of the dancers in the show was the young Bob Fosse, Jack Cole's protégé.

While Davey Burns had years of experience, I was just a kid and theater was a new experience for me. The concepts of upstage and downstage were brand-new. Davey could have easily taken advantage of me. Instead, he couldn't have been more generous. On opening night in New York he turned to me and said, "Sid, if I start to upstage you, you upstage me. If I start to talk loud, you talk louder." He was trying to help.

We did a sketch together where Davey played an old man who refused to give up his spot on the stoop of a brownstone to a film crew shooting a movie in that spot. I played the very British director, while

Davey was criticizing everything we were doing. His character had been in the garment business and had a thick Yiddish accent. Finally, I went over to ask him to leave. He said, "I'm a man who knows my business. When I made a garment, it was not like this piece of fluff." When he began to criticize the costumes, I "lost" my very British accent and in a similar Yiddish accent said, "Look, Mister. What I forgot about garments, you'll never know. That's how I got into the movie business."

With Max's help, I began to create my own material, which we integrated into the show. I played a very honest penny gumball machine in the subway. When I was empty I would try not to take the penny from the customers. After three times of trying to return the penny, I would get beat up by the customer. "So that's how the game is played," I said, and after that kept the pennies without dispensing the gum. The owner of the machine, finding the machine full of pennies and not one gumball missing, marvels at my industriousness and decides that my talent is being wasted in the subway. I am promoted to be a dollar slot machine and moved to Las Vegas.

I also developed a satire on inflation, "The Five Dollar Date," which became one of my signature pieces. It was based on my own dating experiences with Florence. In the first part of the sketch I described the events of an extravagant and romantic night on the town with a girlfriend in Manhattan in 1938, all on just five dollars, going from cab to restaurant to theater to nightclub. It was a time when you could just wink and five cabs would be fighting for you.

In the second part of the sketch, I recreated the same night ten years later, and the result is a miserable night where I deal with rude people, long lines, unpleasant crowds, and a much higher price tag for the night out. The sketch grew to be eight minutes long, a very frenetically paced piece, with me playing all the characters myself to an insistent musical accompaniment — going from cab to theater to restaurant, going from drivers, chefs, and ushers in 1938, effusive over a nickel tip, to the same people not so happy ten years later, and me being rushed, pushed, and called cheap in various incarnations.

Ten years ago, when five dollars was a bankroll, you took your girl out for a big time and the town was really yours. So let us look into the case of a fellow, a girl, a date. The place,

Manhattan. The year, 1938.

"Hello baby. You better get ready. I'm comin' down to do the town to get my steady. We'll do the town and baby we'll rocket. Because I've got five dollars and it's burning a hole in my pocket!"

"We'll taxi to the Le Faize for a dry martini, then we'll taxi to Luigi's for some scallopini, then we'll taxi to the Strand for a picture show, then we'll taxi for chow mein to Foo Yung Bo, then we'll dance and we'll dance. Then a hansom cab through the park. We'll do the town, because I've got five dollars and it's burning a hole in my pocket!"

"Taxi!"

"Yes, sir! Anywhere. Step right in. I'll take you there."

"Here we are."

"A nickel tip. Some tip!"

We are greeted by an effusive maître d' at a French restaurant. He gives the two of us a table reserved for six. We are served martinis out of the crystal glasses. Imported cheese "compliments of the house." I pay the check and tip the waiter.

"Ten cents. Quelle tip!" he exclaims.

"Taxi! To the Strand!"

"At your command!"

"Step right up, seating in all parts of the theater. On the stage, Benny Goodman, Bing Crosby, Bob Hope, Jack Benny, in person. On the screen, we have Clark Gable, Lana Turner, Spencer Tracey, Ingrid Bergman, in Technicolor! And that ain't all! Free dishes, silverware, crockery, china, lounge chairs, screeno, bingo, bango, lotto, a chance to win fifty dollars! All seats twenty-five cents. Free turkeys, free cheese, buy your tickets, please . . ."

"I've got five dollars and I've still got change in my pocket!"

Fast forward to 1948. Same boy, same girl. On the same date:

"Hello baby. You better hurry. Cause it's a worry. We won't be able to get a table. I'm comin' down and I'm comin' fast. I got two months pay, and I hope it will last."

"Taxi!"

"Wherever you're going, I'm not going that way! A dollar tip. Cheapskate!"

"Hello Pierre, you look great."

"Back in the line. Two-hour wait!"

"Let's go to the Strand."

"What's playing?"

"What's the difference? It's a four-hour wait."

"Where's the line?"

"Just keep walking till you find it."

"All we did was fight, fight, fight . . .
What a lousy night! That's a date in
Manhattan today!"

A very physically strenuous piece, "The
Five Dollar Date" pulled together all my
talents — singing, acting, double-talking,
pantomiming.

I wrote the music; Max and I wrote the
lyrics. It was funny and musical and required
technique and dexterity — like Donald
O'Connor in "Make 'Em Laugh," the song
from *Singin' in the Rain*. It was the closing,
the big spot that preceded the finale. It
took a lot of strength to do it eight times a
week.

There were twenty-two pieces in the
revue of *Make Mine Manhattan*. My part
grew to the point where I was in twelve of
the sketches. Comedy sketches were followed
by musical or dance numbers. I also did a
sketch about a diner across the street from
the United Nations, with delegates coming
in to sample the cuisine and use the phone.
That called for different ambassadors, an
Englishman, a Frenchman, a German, a
Persian, and a Russian. I played Hassan

Persha of the Persian delegation ("Father of the moon, son of the stars, cousin of the planets, and brother-in-law of the Milky Way"). My Russian delegate scoffed, "Borscht à la Molotov? That's tomato soup à la Campbell!" Initially, they were going to have different actors playing each nationality. I said I could do all of those guys. And I double-talked all the languages.

No one had ever seen this type of comedy before. Performances began to sell out. The show and I were a big hit. We were very successful in our out-of-town performances in New Haven and Philadelphia. We were making money on the road, which was unusual in the theater business. Joe Hyman became nervous that he could lose his leading man with two weeks' notice. I then renegotiated with Hyman for a much more lucrative deal. I was going to get $1,500 a week and 5 percent of the box office.

During one snowy matinee performance well into the run, I was in the middle of the "Five Dollar Date" and my mind drifted. I began thinking about where I would be eating after the performance. Should I go across the street to Sardis, or should I have a couple of sandwiches sent in from the Gaiety? Because I'd done the number so often, I was almost on automatic pilot. I was fast-talking in a lot of languages, back and forth, when all of a sudden I looked up and didn't know where I was in the number. I looked at Phil, my piano player, who was vamping, the only one who suspected anything might be wrong. And then I looked at the position of my hands, and I was able to remember where I was in the number. The music and the physical movements were so well timed that my hands and my body brought me back to the song. The choreography saved me.

I stayed with the show for a year. New Year's Eve 1948 was my last performance. I won *Billboard*'s coveted Donaldson Award, the equivalent of the Tony, for my performance. Paul Robeson was the first Donaldson Award winner. At the time I didn't even know what the award was. I was replaced by Bert Lahr, who was a great vaudeville and Broadway star, but will always be best known for being the Cowardly Lion in *The Wizard of Oz*.

At the end of my run in *Make Mine Manhattan*, Florence and I took a vacation at the Avon Lodge, and Max went back to Camp Tamiment to work on his shows. When I got back from the mountains, there was a message from Max.

"We're going to have lunch with a fellow from NBC," Max said when I called him back. The fellow was Sylvester "Pat" Weaver, who was vice president in charge of television at NBC. This was 1949, and it was surprising to me that television had reached a level of importance where it had vice presidents.

It was my first meeting and the beginning of a long friendship with one of the giants of television. Pat was one of the few executives who really understood entertainment, not to mention the value of comedians. His brother was comedian Doodles Weaver. Pat wound up creating and producing many great projects, including television institutions like the *Today Show* and *The Tonight Show* — and his daughter, Sigourney Weaver. We went to the Roast Beef House on 52nd Street and I immediately looked at the menu because I was very hungry. Pat, who had been up to Camp Tamiment and had seen Max's productions, said, "Can you do a new show every week?" "Yes," Max confidently replied.

"Well, what do you want? Do you want a half hour, an hour, or an hour and a half?"

I still had food on my mind. "Gee, an hour and a half," I said. "That's a long time to wait for a steak sandwich. An hour, maybe."

And he said, "No. Do you want to do a half hour, an hour, or an hour and a half show?" I had missed the "show" part.

So Max and I looked at each other, and we both said, "Let's do the hour and a half," figuring more was better and not realizing what we had just agreed to. That was it. That's how my television career began.

After Pat left, the reality began to dawn on me. I asked Max, "We're going to write a ninety-minute show every week for thirty-nine weeks?"

Max said, "Hey listen — I think we can do it." He was also nervous. We laughed. If it flopped, who would know? Neither of us knew anyone who owned a television.

The show was going to be fully sponsored by Admiral, a manufacturer of radios and television sets, and would be called *The Admiral Broadway Revue*. The show was being packaged by Max's agent, William Morris.

I was already making up to $3,500 a week performing at the Roxy and the Copa, but I was willing to take a pay cut to work in television. I asked for $1,000 a week, but William Morris wanted to pay me only $900. I reached an impasse with the agent in charge, who told me to take a walk. So I did. The agent went to Max and said, "We have to get another comedian. We have lists of them." Max was beside himself. "The show just walked out the door," he told the agent. "I built the entire show around him. No Caesar, no show." I got the extra hundred dollars.

Max hired the dancers and the singer. When it came to the comedy, he would run all his choices by me for approval. He brought in Mel Tolkin and Lucille Kallen, two very talented young writers he'd worked with at Camp Tamiment. He brought in two actresses — Mary McCarty and a lovely little lady with big brown eyes named Imogene Coca. Imogene and Max also went back to Camp Tamiment. They'd originated *The Straw Hat Revue* with Danny Kaye that eventually went to Broadway. I always called her Immy because she was so little. We had chemistry right away and liked each other immediately. We did one or two sketches together early on, and I didn't even have to think about her timing. We were in sync. Our creative minds both worked the same way.

The production crew was equally impressive. The musical director was Charlie Sanford, who had also been the musical director of *Make Mine Manhattan*. Fred Fox was in charge of set design and Paul Dupont was in charge of costumes. Jimmy Starbuck was the choreographer, and Irwin Kostal was the musical arranger.

The proposed budget was $19,000 a week, meager even by 1949 standards. But Max wanted his foot in the television door. We adopted the format of a Broadway revue. Max's forte was production numbers. He had a lot of experience with music and dance, and his biggest gift was at picking out talent. Although I was the top name on the cast list, I would be in only one or two sketches plus some additional routines or pieces of business here and there.

One of the theaters NBC bought for its fledgling television business was the International Theater on 59th Street off Columbus Circle. It was the theater that William Randolph Hearst built for Gloria Swanson, with whom he had a clandestine affair. There was a private seat all the way at the top of the 1,500-seat theater where Hearst himself would sit to watch the performances.

We were far from the only people to use that theater. At the end of the show, they would move us out and move another program in. NBC would do all kinds of shows from there, and the theater was also let out for musical productions.

We got to the theater at eight o'clock in the morning on February 11, 1949. Our first show was that night. The technicians were walking around with cables, saying things like "You got the male for this, the female for this one?" They didn't know where to put the microphones. There were no body mikes, so they started with fifteen mikes that were placed in the footlights. It didn't do the trick. I came up with the idea of using a retractable boom mike like they did in Hollywood. We had two boom mikes, one for stage left and one for stage right (I knew what those were by now). All the executives worried about was the cost of the four extra men required to operate the boom.

We rehearsed without cameras. We had to wait for the cameras to come in from Ebbets Field or Yankee Stadium. That's how new television was; even cameras had to do double duty. The mechanics were setting up the stage, and the performers were trying on costumes in the empty auditorium. It was hours before show time. The adrenaline was pumping. And everyone was wondering whether it could all happen.

We were kids. It was nervous energy and history all in one. Not only had we never done anything on this grand scale on live television, no one had. Everyone was running around. It was mayhem à la mode.

There was no control room. The only way the director saw us was through three tiny monitors in the dressing room on the second floor. They had no control board. All the buttons and wires connected to the cameras were open and exposed.

Max got up on stage and started to make a speech about what we needed to do and who needed to do what. I looked at Max screaming and getting hoarse. I got up onstage with a bunch of papers, all of which were blank. I thought I would use a little comedy to help break the tension. I handed the papers to Max and said, "Settle this for me. Is this in or out?" pointing to the script. He looked at the empty papers and said, "This is out. Do this number this way." Max was so befuddled he wasn't focusing, he was so nervous he was seeing text on blank pages.

The Admiral Broadway Revue was broadcast live on both NBC and the old Dumont network. (At the time, the coaxial cable went only as far as Chicago. West of that, shows were recorded on kinescopes and rebroadcast a week later.) The premiere episode was virtually one long commercial for the sponsor's products — refrigerators, ranges, phonographs, and "magic mirror television." As the theme song said, "Bringing the top of entertainment for you, trying to bring Broadway into your home." It was the first time a home entertainment system, an integrated television, phonograph, and radio, was ever displayed on television, and it was available for $399. We even did a sketch live right in one of their stores.

On the first show I reprised the sketch from *Make Mine Manhattan* about the United Nations. Radio comedian Roy Atwood did a long commercial for all the Admiral products. I did the "Five Dollar Date" number for the first time on television. I also did a parody of the opera *Carmen* with Imogene.

Other than a couple of small mistakes, the show went off well. More important, the people loved it. We were an overnight hit. When I walked down the street people said, "Hello, Sid." Someone was watching.

During rehearsals for the Admiral show, Mel Brooks sometimes came to the International Theater. He would make catlike noises and scratch at the door in order to be let in. My manager, Leo Pillot, refused to believe that Mel knew me, and had two ushers grab him and literally toss him into the alley. When I found out about it, I told them that we were friends and it was okay to let him in.

I remember introducing Mel to Max. Mel would do a little song where he would get down on one knee, which he did for Max:

Here I am, I'm Melvin Brooks,
I've come to stop the show,
Just a ham who's minus looks,
But in your hearts I'll grow.
I'll tell ya gags, I'll sing you songs,
Just happy little snappy tunes that roll along.
I'm out of my mind, so won't you be kind,
And please love . . . Melvin Brooks!

Max looked at me and said, "Who is this meshuggener?" — Yiddish for "crazy person." He didn't know how right he was.

The show ran on Friday nights, for nineteen weeks, from February to June 1949. I thought we were doing well, both critically and with the audience, and suddenly Admiral withdrew its sponsorship. I couldn't believe it; we were doing very well, but we were canceled. It didn't make any sense.

It was only after the season that I learned the truth. That summer I had a two-week engagement at the Chicago Theater, where I was held over for eight weeks. I got a phone call from Ross Siragusa, the president of Admiral. He invited me to come over and have lunch with him. "I think I owe you an explanation as to why the *Admiral Broadway Revue* was canceled." I will never forget him telling me that the show was so popular that Admiral could not keep up with the demand for television sets that the program generated. When the show first began, Admiral had been producing fifty to a hundred sets a week, and selling the same number. The popularity of the show caused business to pick up, and within months orders skyrocketed to 5,000 sets a *day*. He was beyond what he could produce.

The company was faced with a choice: it could continue to sponsor the show, or it could take that money and build a new factory. Siragusa told me that they had decided to build the new factory, and that's why the show was killed. "You mean the show was too good?" I asked. "Yes," he said. "It was a little too rich for our blood." The *Admiral Broadway Revue* was and is probably the only show in history to be canceled because it was too successful.

Part 2
THE GOLDEN DECADE

Chapter 6

YOUR SHOW OF SHOWS
AND CAESAR'S HOUR

The late 1940s and early 1950s were a magical time. The war was over. We were happy to be alive. And we were grateful. There was a feeling of hope and opportunity that permeated the country. There was the sense that anything was attainable if you were willing to work hard enough for it.

It wasn't at all like the Great Depression, where you had homeless people living in Hoovervilles because the government didn't help anyone. Almost 8 million veterans received educational benefits via the GI bill. The GI Bill was the best move the government ever made. Guys came out of the service and not only went to school; they came out and got married right away. They all needed homes, and you could get a GI loan for that. Despite an escalating Cold War, there was a feeling of optimism.

People were busy with their own lives. We even shrugged off the money we loaned to Britain, France, and Russia to fight World War II, hundreds of millions of dollars. We spend that much now on iced tea.

Walking around New York City, you could feel a tangible electricity in the air. Men all wore suits and ties. Women wore hats and gloves and dresses. People's shoes were polished. There was a sense of style and elegance.

There was a restaurant called the Brass Rail on Broadway, where a chef with a white uniform and a big white hat would stand in the window and carve a standing prime rib like he was playing the cello. He was an artist.

I used to dream about Radio City, which I thought of as a working museum because of its gorgeous 1920s Art Deco style. As a kid I had gone down there with my class to see *Little Women* with Katharine Hepburn. I now walked by it almost every day. The Roxy and Capitol theaters, with their marble staircases, were modern-day palaces. It was a buck and a half to go to the movies for two at night. The divans, big love seats, were major splurges at $1.25 each. That was high class.

Every new advance was greeted with a

sense of wonderment and excitement. It was a big thing when a new car came out and there were new clothing styles every fall. You needed to put your name on a list to get a car — any car. For a long time new cars came in either black or black. The two-toned Oldsmobile was a big deal. The little MG Roadster was very popular. And there was this new invention, television, that was starting to blossom at the same time I was. Everything I'd done up to that point — the Catskills, the Coast Guard, being a musician and a Broadway actor — had been, without my knowing it, part of my preparation for television. Television offered the opportunity for writers and artists to collaborate. The canvas was the little black box that projected images into thousands and later millions of living rooms all over the country.

The corpse of the *Admiral Broadway Revue* wasn't cold, and Max and Pat Weaver were planning our return to television. Pat was now executive vice president in charge of television at NBC, and the wheels of the mind that would create the *Today Show* and *The Tonight Show* were turning rapidly.

The goal was amazingly ambitious yet very simple, starting with the fact that people go out on Saturday night to be entertained. If you offered them the same entertainment opportunity on television, they wouldn't have to spend a lot of money. They wouldn't even have to leave their living rooms. People were starved for entertainment and it came into your home. That's why I always liked the idea of TV — you don't have to worry about dinner, parking, tipping the headwaiter, getting caught in the rain, or catching a cab to the theater. All you had to do was turn on your set.

The financial lesson from the Admiral experience — the only time in television history that a show was canceled for being too popular — was that no one sponsor could carry an hour and a half show of this magnitude alone.

In 1949 advertising executives and the networks were barely comfortable with the business of radio. Television was an entirely new industry, a novelty — a picture came into your home with sound. No one knew how long it would last, or for that matter whether it would last at all.

The logistics of television were a maze. Networks were little more than facilities for the advertisers to use to broadcast the shows they created, owned, and controlled.

It was not only more challenging than

radio, but much more expensive. The prevailing mind-set at the time was to have the sponsor's name over the name of the show, which made the concept of multiple sponsorships all the more difficult to sell.

The one-sponsor concept worked in radio because all you needed was a studio, seats, and a couple of microphones, music stands, and a script. There was no scenery, no crew to run through quick and elaborate set changes, no makeup, props, costumes, numerous extras, and all the other things that were required for a major television production. You could sponsor an entire radio show for $15,000 per episode and cover all of the costs. Jack Benny, Fred Allen, and Burns and Allen cost $19,000 each. That was pocket change compared to the $64,000 that *Your Show of Shows* eventually cost.

Milton Berle was a key figure in this transition. He brought the vaudeville format to television, which was a monumental achievement and opened many doors for other entertainers, including myself. Milton was crucial to the development of our format because he showed the networks that a new show could be done every week. He also demonstrated that audiences were willing to tune in to the same performers every week in the variety context. The difference in the format made Milton's show much less expensive to produce than ours. There was less scenery required. They were all guest acts that all brought their own costumes. So Milton's sponsor could afford the cost of his show.

What Pat Weaver proposed was two shows, two and a half hours of comedy, which would air consecutively on Saturday nights from 8:00 to 10:30. That would keep the audiences in their homes. Pat developed the concept of a magazine show so that you didn't need a single sponsor to carry it. There were to be several different sponsors. He proposed that the shows have rotating commercials, which would guarantee every sponsor at least one exposure during each half hour segment. At the time, though, most cities only had one or two channels, which were allowed to pick and choose what they wanted to air from each of the networks. They could even show only one half hour of a variety show that ran an hour or an hour and a half. So if a city didn't air a half hour block, the sponsor would have to get a refund. The FCC didn't approve the plan, so sponsors had to choose one half hour segment within which to advertise.

Pat put his head on the block because he had no sponsors ready to step up. He got NBC and its parent company, RCA, to foot the costs for the first few shows. We waited four weeks before we could get sponsors. Pat was taking a big risk that, fortunately, paid off for all of us.

Until that time, the only big things on television were bowling, wrestling, and Charlie Chan. Television comedy consisted of mostly burlesque sketches. Max's plan from the beginning was that the new show was not going to be a repeat of the *Admiral Broadway Revue*. It was going to be grander and more ambitious.

We set out to innovate television, which was an evolving medium in its infancy. Our first conception was to deliver to the audience the first act of a Broadway show. It was an hour and a half long, with tickets and a playbill. Most of the audience had never seen live entertainment. Even today, the vast majority of the people in this country will never see live entertainment outside of sports, large musical concerts, or a comedy club.

There would be no more weekly theme the way there was in the Admiral show. Instead, there would be a different guest host each week who would open the show and participate in new and original sketches and musical numbers. The plan was to have two new original sketches in each half hour. This may sound routine now, but at the time it was out there on the cutting edge.

Max also envisioned including operatic numbers, ballets, and soloists in the new show. He wasn't interested in the American public's lowest common denominator. He wasn't going to dumb down, he was going to lift up. Taste, class, and style were going to be the order of the day. Max's goal was that the quality of the show would drive its popularity and ultimately elevate taste.

This was going to be Max's crowning moment, the culmination of everything he learned and wanted to do in thirty years in show business. The program was going to be called, optimistically and somewhat arrogantly, *Your Show of Shows*.

Max was putting the new team together and hiring the comedy troupe, but he would again run all his choices by me for approval. He'd noticed I'd worked very well with Imogene Coca and I loved the idea of teaming up with her again. We hadn't had a lot to do together during the short run of the *Admiral Broadway Revue*, but when we did, we really clicked. It was a symbiotic thing that I can't explain to this day.

I was a very physical comedian and I needed a sidekick who was not only funny but was a person I could pick up with one hand. When Howard Morris first came in to audition, I reached out, grabbed him by the lapels, lifted him up, and did the scene. I turned to Max and said, "I think he's going to be okay." We did a sketch together early on where I was the violin teacher and Howie was the student. Howie was supposed to have an aluminum plate hidden under a wig, but he forgot to put it on. "No, no, no! Not like that." I took the bow out of his hand. Each no was followed by a rap on the head with the bow. I kept whacking him on the head, and after a few of my shots he started to go down. I realized he didn't have the plate on and I had to ad-lib right away. So I grabbed him and waltzed off the stage. "That's your lesson for today," I said. Howie went right with it. He was game for anything and became a core member of the troupe.

Howie and Mel Brooks also became fast friends. When Howie first came on board, Max introduced him to the writers: Mel Tolkin, Lucille Kallen, and a little Frenchman named "Monsieur Bri," who

Max said was researching American television. For the next two days, Monsieur Bri said very little to Howie. When he did speak, it was in broken French, which was laced with what sounded suspiciously like Yiddish. On the third day, Monsieur Bri walked up to Howie, extended his hand, losing the French accent, and said, "Howie, how the hell are you?"

Despite their friendship, Howie became, like everyone else, a victim of Mel's insanity. Just before one Christmas, Howie and Mel were leaving rehearsal at the City Center. At the bottom of the stairs, Mel turned to Howie and said, "Stick 'em up." Howie said "What are you doing," which only made Mel angrier: "Shut up, give me everything you got! EVERYTHING!!" So Howie gave Mel his watch, his wedding ring, his wallet, his driver's license. In short, everything. Mel gave it all back the next day as a Christmas gift.

The following year, history and Mel repeated themselves. Howie and Mel were in a rowboat in the pond in Central Park, and as Howie rowed under a bridge, Mel said, "Give me your wallet, or I'll throw you in the water and drown you." Mel was so crazy, you had to believe him, so Howie gave up all his valuables. Howie then took off his shoes, stepped out of the boat into the three-feet deep water, and walked back to shore. Mel again gave everything back the following Christmas as a gift. The holidays meant a lot to him.

We also needed a straight man. Making that choice tough was the fact that Max subscribed to the comedy tradition that the straight man had to be taller than the comedian. Since I was six feet one that led to a succession of people Max would flatly dismiss because they literally didn't measure up. He would regretfully tell a fine actor of only five feet eleven what a shame it was that he wasn't just a few inches taller, that he couldn't be stretched on the rack just a few more inches.

Carl Reiner had starred in a competing CBS show, *The 54th Street Revue*. He was also a successful Broadway actor in shows like *Call Me Mister* and *Pretty Penny*, which was directed by George S. Kaufman. When Carl's latest show, a revue called *Alive and Kicking*, developed problems, who else but Max Liebman was brought in as a play doctor. The first thing he asked Carl was, "How tall are you?" The rest is history.

Carl was an immediate success. He was a comedian himself, and he truly understood and still understands comedy. Most people still don't realize the importance of a straight man in comedy, or how difficult that role is. Carl had to make his timing my timing. He is an amazing performer and is the best straight man I've ever worked with.

On the physical side of production, Max was able to bring back most of the crew from the *Admiral Broadway Revue*, including Charlie Sanford as the musical director and Irwin Kostal, who won an Emmy for his musical arrangements.

Freddy Fox came back as the set designer, a really critical position. We created all our own stock sets, which I called the Polish hall because they reminded me of the old Polish community center where I had played gigs as a teenager. Each set piece was numbered and color-coded and stored in a warehouse in Brooklyn. Sets are very important. They have to surround the performer with as much atmosphere as possible without getting in the way of the performance.

The stagehands, the people who had to deal with all those sets, loved the show. They would take short naps in the afternoon so that they could be fresh and sharp for show time. We had different colored pieces of tape on the floor and the walls to match the scenery, which was broken down and stacked and then rebuilt and replaced. They could go from full stage to full stage in a minute and ten seconds, which had never been done before. They adopted the United States Marines slogan: "The difficult we can do now, the impossible may take a little longer."

Our choreographer, Jimmy Starbuck, had to do at least three big production numbers a week, and at least two smaller ones. He was not only the most prolific choreographer, he was the most creative. Ed Herlihy was the show's announcer, a lovely and giving man with a great voice.

On the musical side of things, Aaron Levine was the manager of the orchestra and the NBC liaison. He was also in charge of making the trains run on time. If you needed a prop, or a costume, or a sandwich, Aaron was the guy you called and he took care of it. He made sure everyone on the show was comfortable. The Billy Williams Quartet was another staple musical component. That was significant because they were black, which was something new at the time for this or any kind of show, but Max was color-blind and quality obsessed.

Your Show of Shows premiered on Saturday night, February 25, 1950, at nine o'clock as part of the *NBC Saturday Night Revue*. Television was still following the radio pattern of launching new shows at the beginning of the year. They didn't know any better at the time, but they later learned that during the summer people went away and didn't take their television sets with them. Even people who stayed at home spent more time outside, which is why ratings would drop off precipitously in July and August. That's also why less expensive summer shows replaced the more costly winter programming.

The original plan was for us to be part of a two-and-a-half-hour block. The first hour, starting at eight o'clock, was a revue that was hosted by my good friend, the comedian Jack Carter. Jack was New York based, but because of the shortage of theater space available in New York City for television use, that show emanated from Chicago. Unfortunately, Jack's show only lasted for one season. As *Your Show of Shows* became a hit, the network favored us and gave Jack a hard time. If Jack's group started to do something similar to what we were doing, like a movie satire, they would cut it, severely limiting Jack and company in what they could do creatively.

Needless to say, there was nervousness

and excitement the entire week before the debut show. Though the coaxial cable went only as far as Chicago and the rest of the country got the shows via kinescope the following week, it was still live and was going out to millions of people. More importantly, this was our second go-round. We never forgot that the *Admiral Broadway Revue* had been a hit and was still canceled!

So there was no guarantee that we would succeed even if we were terrific. No one had ever done this before; there was no rulebook or history we could draw on. Circumstances beyond our control could once again knock us off the air. Who knew how many chances we would have after that. Talk about pressure!

The premiere began with the theme song, "Stars over Broadway" (written by Mel Tolkin). Burgess Meredith was the guest host and Gertrude Lawrence was a guest star. Lily Pons sang and Mischa Elman performed a violin solo. Robert Merrill sang on the show. It was the first time opera was performed on a television comedy show by a professional opera singer. He performed an excerpt from *La Traviata* with Marguerite Piazza. Max once said that he had been doing television all of his life, just without the cameras. The cameras were now there, and he was a success. He really pulled it together with style and class, and it gave me something to play off against.

As soon as we saw the audience reaction, we knew we were a hit. We didn't have to wait for the critics — the audience will tell you how you're doing every time. No matter what technological advances the future brings, to a performer there will probably never be anything more euphoric or exhilarating than a grateful audience showing its appreciation with applause and standing ovations during a live performance.

Still, the reviews, when they came, were excellent. Alfred Hitchcock wrote that "Caesar best approaches the young Charlie Chaplin of the early 1920s." John Crosby of the *New York Herald Tribune* (and a radio and television critic who was not known for his kind words) wrote, "Sid Caesar is one of the wonderments of the modern electronic age." He also wrote that "Sid Caesar has more genuinely funny comedy sequences than he knows what to do with," that his routines "are even funnier the second time," and "that he has restored the art of pantomime to the high estate it enjoyed before the talkies and radio."

With this show, unlike the Admiral show,

I was sensitive to how we were doing in the ratings. We were consistently in the top three slots. We were a significant force in America on Saturday nights in the early 1950s. Families made watching the show an event. To this day, I still get people who come up to me and say, "Thank you for the laughter of my childhood." When people remember the shows, they not only remember the comedy, they remember their parents, grandparents, brothers, sisters, aunts, and uncles. They remember a time when everyone was together and everyone was laughing. There were no arguments, squabbles, or fights. Whatever was going on at home, for at least an hour and a half on Saturday night, people got to laugh and they got to see their parents laugh, and they have that memory to hold on to. I feel honored to have given them that. I may be missing something, but I don't think there is one show today that an entire family gets together to watch.

From 9:00 to 10:30, we had a Broadway revue. The show was a fertile training ground for future Broadway playwrights, as evidenced by Mike Stewart, who went on to write *Hello Dolly* and *Bye Bye Birdie*; Joe Stein, who wrote *Fiddler on the Roof*; Larry Gelbart, whose works include *A*

Funny Thing Happened on the Way to the Forum and *Mastergate*; Carl Reiner, who wrote *Enter Laughing*; Woody Allen, who wrote *Play It Again, Sam* and *Don't Drink the Water*; Neil Simon, who wrote practically everything else; and most recently Mel Brooks, who fifty years later delivered Broadway one of its greatest hits, in *The Producers*. As of 2001, Mel is only one of two people in history to win an Oscar, an Emmy, a Tony, and a Grammy.

The key to the success of the show was very simple, if not amazingly challenging to execute week after week — we had the ability to extract humor out of everyday life. The humor sprang from everyday events and was a mixture of the sad and funny. The guy in trouble is a very funny guy. Chaplin knew that in 1910 and we knew that in 1950. You have to be emotionally invested and involved with and worried about the guy you're going to laugh at or cry with. If you like the character you're watching on the screen, you'll be interested in him. If you don't, you'll either change the channel or turn off the set.

In the beginning there was just Max, myself, Mel Tolkin, and Lucille Kallen writing the show, with Mel Brooks pitching ideas without officially being part of the staff. I was paying Mel out of my own pocket. The success or failure of the show now rested squarely on my shoulders. My name was on the top of the show, and that drove both my thought processes and my anxieties. Initially, though, there was nothing for even me to be anxious about. The show was so popular that Broadway show receipts were down on Saturday night, and so were restaurants and taxi-cabs. A group of Broadway movie-house owners went to an NBC executive and begged him to use his influence to get *Your Show of Shows* rescheduled for a time slot during the week. A dead night, like Thursday. It never happened.

What did happen was that Imogene and I became television's royal couple in the early 1950s. There was a popular joke out there at the time that the fans themselves made up. It went: "Why didn't Imogene Coca take a bath?" "Because Sid 'sees her.'" When Immy and I were honored at the Polo Grounds before a game, thousands of people started chanting the punch line. If you're on television every week, people welcome you into their living rooms or bedrooms, and they feel that they know you. A lot of people thought Imogene and I were married to each other. Once I was at a party with Florence and a woman looked askance at my tall and statuesque wife and said, "I wonder if Imogene knows about her." "She certainly does," I told her. "That's my *real* wife."

Soon after we became a hit, Max came to me and suggested that Imogene's name be elevated to the top of the show next to mine. I immediately agreed. "She deserves it," I told him. I remember how both pleased and proud Max was at my unequivocal response.

For two people who could not have been more different, Imogene and I were creatively and instinctively connected. Immy anticipated me. She gave me the ability to think, and the ability to put more into the sketches. Katharine Hepburn and Spencer Tracy made music together on screen, but I was twice as lucky. I not only had Imogene, afterward I had Nanette Fabray. Immy and I did not talk much offstage, but when we hit that stage it was as if we were one person. Working with her was like working with somebody you'd known your entire life from moment one. There was a genuineness and an authenticity that was built on an emotional foundation. We protected each other. Our instincts and timing were so well aligned that it was as if

Imogene knew exactly what I was thinking. We would allow each other opportunities to run with moments and lines and do pieces of business. I didn't have to worry about her timing, whether she was going to come in at the right time or not. We were in sync. No matter where we ran, we always came back with the cue. To a comedic performer, to have that kind of support is more valuable than anything else. Our minds both worked the same way. There's no name for it; it just happened.

In an interview years later Immy said, "You know what I wish for most in the world? That Sid and I could work together again. I'd run twenty miles in sheer joy. It was the most fulfilling time in my life. We are alike in so many ways. I'd take fifty bucks a week for the chance to work with him again." I felt the same way.

All this success meant that Pat Weaver was also able to breathe easier. Within a few weeks, he had sold all of the show's commercial time for the entire thirty-nine weeks. The sponsors were lining up and probably at a much higher rate than they would have paid had they sold at the beginning before the show started. After the spots, we were left with twenty-six and a half minutes per half hour. That's as opposed to today's nineteen minutes per half hour with eleven minutes of commercials. That change in the commercial structure over the years is what drove my reluctance to ever offer the shows up for commercial syndication. That's seven minutes of commercial per hour. During the hour and a half, we had seventy-nine and a half minutes of show. Someone with either no experience, or someone with no regard for the comedy, would cut it down tremendously and unwittingly ruin it.

One of the true personal symbols of my own early success has to do with man's eternal love affair with the convertible. It started, classically, on a dark and rainy night in 1951, with me driving home from the Copacabana nightclub with Florence. We were still living in Queens at the time, and when I drove over the 59th Street Bridge, the tires got caught in the trolley tracks and we swerved and crashed into one of the concrete pillars.

The first thing I did was to make sure that Florence was all right. Because of the rain, we had only been traveling about fifteen miles an hour, so we weren't hurt. The car, however, was pretty banged up. Fortunately, within seconds a guy was there with a tow truck and a cab was waiting. It was like they choreographed it. I could tell that they had done this before. "Give us your car, Mr. Caesar," I was told, "and we'll take care of everything."

The next morning I called my brother Dave in Yonkers. I told him about the accident and then I said, "Dave, do you remember the convertible we saw in the window at the Cadillac dealership?" "Sure," he said. "Could you buy it for me and drive it over? I'll drive you back home."

I could almost see Dave smiling over the phone. He was almost as excited about my getting a convertible as I was. "Sure, Sid. I could do that. I'll be passing Weber's Bakery on my way over. How about a dozen rolls with the car?"

What I bought was a black Cadillac convertible with a red leather interior and whitewall tires. It was the first convertible with the windscreen in the back seat that swiveled up so that women could sit without their hair flying around. That in my mind was a real rite of passage: I was no longer a working stiff. Because of what it meant to me, I held on to that car for a long time.

When *Your Show of Shows* became a hit, we started to make money, and I started to tip very well. Actually I used to overtip. In the era of the $2 tip, I would give away as much as $20 to the headwaiter at Danny's Hideaway, where the writers and I would all get together every week after the show. I also developed a taste for good Havana cigars. Up the block from the City Center there was a cigar store. In the window there was a humidor with fifty cigars. There were market selection Churchill cigars, which were especially made for Winston Churchill. When I smoked those cigars, I felt like the king of England. The taste and aroma were captivating. I bought a box of fifty and I took them home. Like Queen Victoria, Florence was not amused. "You spent $50 on cigars?" she said in disbelief. "Florence," I said, "we make more than $50." The little luxuries went a long way.

A not-so-little luxury was the suits we all bought. I made a lot of tailors rich by ordering handmade suits with the broadest possible padded shoulders. At one point I had about a hundred of them. In those days, people got dressed up to go to work and I wore a suit, cuff links, and gold collar stays (which obviously only I knew about) to the office every day. It was part of establishing my authority. Though what it did to my authority to sit around in my shorts, which I did on hot days so my pants wouldn't get creased, I'm not sure. We all showed off our suits in the office because with our hectic schedule we weren't going anywhere else.

Having money meant that both Max and I moved to Park Avenue, but with a difference. Max hired a private chef to cook for him and ran with "the chichi crowd," while I ran with "the boys." I always remembered where I came from. When Dave first came to visit me at my apartment on Park Avenue and 81st Street, we took a walk outside and I started to light a cigar. Dave smiled and asked, "Is it all right to smoke on Park Avenue?"

On Sundays, Dave would come over with my mother and Abe. Often Fat Jackie Leonard, a very brilliant comedian, would come by with cheesecake in hand. I'd buy enough Nova salmon and sturgeon for everyone, even at $5 a pound.

Because I burned off a lot of energy on the sketches, I always ate a lot. For breakfast I would have orange juice, steak and eggs, applesauce, even potatoes. Lunch would be at least one pastrami sandwich. For dinner, I would eat a lobster, then a thick cut of prime rib with a saddle on it,

181

with mushrooms and maybe a jockey thrown in.

I did have one particular weakness: New York hot dogs. Once I was in a limo with the writers and I saw a hot dog vendor on the corner of Sixth Avenue pushing a small cart with an umbrella over it. We stopped immediately. The vendor saw a group of men in big hats and overcoats pull up suddenly and jump out of the car. The poor guy was terrified. He thought we were gangsters. "Take what you want!" he said. "No," I said, "all I need is some mustard and sauerkraut."

I loved Italian food and Cantonese food. We used to go to Little Italy and Chinatown for meals. We had soup and hors d'oeuvres in one restaurant and then the main course in a fine Italian restaurant that made the best marinara sauce, with the chauffeur following us as we walked from one place to the other. There was one dessert place that we always ended up at.

Another new luxury was golf. I took up the game in 1951. By my tenth or twelfth game I had learned how to hold a club. By my twentieth round I had been invited to a tournament at the Lake Success Golf Club in Kings Point, Long Island, with Dean Martin (who was an excellent golfer), Jerry Lewis, Perry Como, Dagmar, and Corinne

Calvet. Hundreds of people lined up in a narrow alleyway to watch me tee off. At the time I could hit a ball 300 yards, but don't ask me where it would go. I would slice the ball and it would wind up in someone's backyard. I started hitting with a driver and then played it safe with a seven iron, looking for both distance and some accuracy.

I would also go shooting in the mountains with my two best friends, Harry Rudetsky, who owned the Joyvah Halvah Company, and Milt Chasen. Harry would have some cans of halvah vacuum packed with water and we would go up to the Avon Lodge and use them for targets. We would set up the cans at 100 and 200 yards against a sand mountain (so there wouldn't be any ricochets if we missed) and we would shoot .220 Rocket rifles and .375 Weatherby Magnums at them. When the bullets hit the cans, the cans exploded. Harry, Milton, and I would play pinochle together and smoke cigars for hours and just talk and laugh. They both loved cigars as much as I did. Recently I lost both of my dear friends, Harry and Milton. They lived their lives well and will be sorely missed.

In 1951 I began a lifelong friendship

with another great comedian with a very fast mind named Buddy Hackett. Right up to the day before he passed away in June 2003, Buddy would call me almost every day just to tell me a joke that he had just made up and make me laugh. Years ago, he would join Milton, Harry, and myself in the mountains. He was up at the Concord Hotel, which was only five miles from the Avon Lodge. He knew a shortcut to the lodge and would come shooting with us. Instead of a rifle, he would shoot with a little .38-caliber pistol. When he hit one of the little cans, I playfully goaded him: "Lucky lucky." He smiled and said "Lucky, lucky? Looky, looky!" He aimed his little gun, cocked it, fired, and hit another can. We all were trained to shoot in the military. Buddy will also be missed, not only by me, but also by everyone that he touched and by anyone who loved to laugh.

It was during that time I met and be-friended a brilliant man by the name of Steve Allen, who was the first host of *The Tonight Show*. He was a talented comedian, composer, and author. I called Steve the Renaissance Man. There wasn't a subject he could not speak intelligently and passionately about. I miss his friendship, his wit, and his wise and thoughtful insights.

Florence and I took the family and our housekeeper, Marinee, who was with us for over forty years, to the Lido Beach Hotel in Atlantic Beach for a few summers. I remember renting a Jaguar, a twelve-cylinder two-seater. It was so powerful, I was afraid to put it in first gear. One summer, I played a few games of tennis with Pancho Gonzales at the Atlantic Beach hotel. The only time I saw the ball was when I served.

In 1954 I met one of my idols, Paul Muni. I remember watching him on the screen as a kid. I was so moved, I could barely speak when we shook hands on the boardwalk. This was Emile Zola! A small crowd had gathered around us. I told him what a big fan I was. "I know who you are," he told me. "I'm a fan of yours too." He was shy, like me. He was a lovely man. We had a mutual admiration society going on.

Success meant that awards followed in clusters for me, the cast, crew, and the production itself. In 1950 Imogene and I were on the *Kate Smith Show* to get an award for being the best comedians of the year. I won my first Emmy on February 18, 1952, the same day my son Rick was born. Cartoonist Al Capp, who created the classic *Lil Abner* comic strip, was also a guest on the show. He used me as a model for one of the strip's characters. Sam Centaur (note the similarity of the name) was based on yours truly. I posed for it with no shirt on. I was also invited to pose for Philippe Halsman, one of the "world's ten greatest photographers," whose images form a vivid picture of prosperous American society in the mid-twentieth century. The whole world was my candy store. Whatever I wanted was there for me, which was all too often a mixed blessing.

One experience of fame I'll never forget happened a few years later, when my daughter Michele was about four years old.

We were living in an apartment building on Long Island at the time. One Sunday morning, Michele was playing with her friends in another apartment downstairs, and they were talking about our show from the night before and a routine I had done. She ran out of her friend's apartment, took the elevator back up to our floor, and rang the doorbell of our apartment.

Sunday morning was the only morning of the week I could sleep late. I woke up to the doorbell and staggered over to the door to see who it was. I opened the door and looked straight ahead. I didn't see anyone there and was about to close the door when I heard a little voice say, "Daddy?" I looked down and saw my daughter. I invited her to come in.

"What's your name?" she asked.

I said, "Daddy."

"What does Mommy call you?"

"She calls me Sidney."

"But do people call you Sid?"

"Yeah, some people."

"And our last name is Caesar?"

"That's right."

I watched the look of realization come over my child's face. "You're Sid Caesar!"

I was even famous in my own home.

At the end of the third season of *Your Show of Shows*, my contract with NBC expired. Florence and I were going by cruise ship to Europe on a nine-week vacation tour. By the time of our bon voyage party on board the *Liberte*, I hadn't signed a new one yet, although NBC had renewed the show for the following season.

Suddenly what seemed like all the lawyers for NBC walked into the stateroom with Pat Weaver. The NBC executives kept presenting numbers on checks they had prepared and were showing them to me. "How about this number?" they'd ask hopefully. "That's not the right number," I said, giving the check back to them. "We'll make up the rest to you." Each time they made an offer, my lawyers and I would go into the bathroom of the stateroom to discuss it. That's where the deal was made. They agreed to my number, which was $25,000 per week. I signed and we sailed.

While we were on the ship to Paris, Columbia Pictures cabled. They wanted me to do a picture with Judy Holliday. They offered to pay for the entire cruise over and above my salary. But thirty-nine hour-and-a-half shows made me a little crazy. "I have to have some diversion," I told them, passing on the opportunity. "I gotta have a rest."

Paris, unfortunately, wasn't restful for me at the time. We were touring from one old church to the next older church, to relics, to stones, to rocks. All of a sudden I had to be places. It felt too much like work. My breaking point was when we were given tickets to go to the Grand Prix in Longchamps outside of Paris. Florence and I were driven there in a limousine. Although everything had supposedly been arranged in advance, no one knew who we were when we got there. Unable to speak French, we couldn't even find our seats.

"Florence," I said, "let's go home." She thought I meant the hotel. "No," I said. "Home." I called TWA and the next morning we were on a plane back to New York. Those were the days when traveling first class meant first-class style. There were real seats with room to stretch and tablecloths and silverware. They served a standing prime rib and bottles of top-shelf liquor. There was a little piano at the front of the plane and Andre Kostelanetz played for us.

Whenever I would get on a plane, I would be invited into the cockpit and pictures would be taken of me at the controls. In case that makes you nervous, I will go on record now as never having piloted a commercial plane.

When we got back, we got in the car and went up to the Concord Hotel in the Catskills. It was just a comfortable environment, unstructured and relaxed. I could decide whether I wanted to go downstairs to eat or have my breakfast in our suite. That was my idea of a vacation.

At my new salary of $25,000 a week for thirty-nine weeks a year, I was making more money than the president, not to mention more money than Clark Gable and other major movie stars. And remember, this was a time when $5 still went a very long way. That got the attention of General David Sarnoff, the head of the RCA Corporation, which owned NBC. He invited me to a private lunch.

General Sarnoff had a huge office at the top of the RCA building in Rockefeller Center that looked like it was right out of a movie set. He had his own private dining room with his own chef and waiter. He sat at the head of the table and I sat next to him.

Halfway through lunch, the general looked at me and said, "You know, Mr. Caesar, you make more in one week than my top engineer makes in a year. A man who studied and has gone to college and graduate school."

"General Sarnoff," I said, meeting fire with fire, "may I put it this way. If you had a tank that had the best chunk of armor that could be built, nothing could pass through it. If you had a gun, a .155-millimeter cannon, which is the biggest gun you could put in a tank, you would have tremendous firepower. The tank would be capable of traveling at a speed of eighty-five miles per hour over any kind of terrain. Think of it — a tank that has all this capability. But if there's nobody there to drive the tank, it's just a piece of iron."

"A driver I can always get," he said.

"Ah, but can he shoot, too?"

The general looked at me in wonderment and asked, "What else would you like to eat?" deftly changing the subject. He didn't know how to respond to that, and he had to let it go. Or maybe he didn't want to get into an argument with the help. Like all straight, solid businessmen, General Sarnoff didn't understand or want to understand artistic attitude. The network executives also didn't want to understand it and they didn't know how to handle it. With *Your Show of Shows*, all of us, especially NBC and Sarnoff, got lucky.

They happened to get a show where everything fit together. The main thing was that the chemistry was right between everyone associated with the project. And where there was chemistry, there was magic. Too many times in the past fifty years networks have put together the best writers, producers, directors, and actors and spent millions of dollars on sets and special effects. The only thing that they were missing was the chemistry among all those players. They wound up with near misses and expensive flops.

A lot of credit for this kind of chemistry has to go to Max, a man who knew what he wanted. He knew talent, and he knew how to put on a show with class and style. In any endeavor in life, you not only need a great teacher but you have to be willing to learn. As I've mentioned before, Max wasn't a teacher in the conventional sense. You learned from Max by watching and studying what he did and what he didn't do.

I already had the knowledge of music, and I could tell if it was a good orchestration or not, but with Max I learned about getting the chorus together, seeing if the songs were done well, if the orchestrations worked in the context of the show, and if the lighting was right. You have to have a wide body of knowledge to make everything come off effectively. I was very eager to learn all of these things.

The art that is never truly appreciated is the running order, which could make or break a variety show. Max had perfected it. "Start with your medium sketch, follow it with something soft and then go into a more powerful number." He would always say: "Never put two big sketches together. They get compared and cancel each other out." I learned a lot from him. I knew a lot about show business at the time, but under Max I learned about how to put on a television show. Max also showed me the importance of how you present and surround a show and how you layer the comedy, especially when you're doing a revue. If you skimp on costs, with cheap costumes and lousy choreography, it takes away from the comedy. Max's productions would go for fourteen or fifteen choruses, which meant you sang for two choruses and then you danced for two more, and then you followed with four or five more songs. You sang and danced and then you danced and sang, and then you sang standing still. You get the idea. That type of staging was his forte.

Experience is the best teacher of all and Max had the experience. He was the coach who knew how to develop his players, maximize their talent, and play into their strengths. He was the doctor who had seen the ailment, could identify all of the symptoms, and know immediately how to treat or fix whatever you had.

As *Your Show of Shows* became more successful, Max added to the roster on every front. He added more musicians and artists. In addition to Marguerite Piazza and the Billy Williams Quartet, there were the dance teams of Mata and Hari, and Bambi Lynn and Rod Alexander. More importantly for me, he brought in more writers. Max and I both believed that writing was the key to the success of the show, and the show's writers were the highest paid in the industry. After we became a hit, the writers were getting paid $2,500 a week.

Max also made sure we had interesting and popular guest stars. These included Dave Garroway, Charlton Heston, Geraldine Page, Arlene Francis, Rex Harrison, Ralph Bellamy, Douglas Fairbanks Jr., Paul Winchell and Jerry Mahoney, Pearl Bailey, and Fred Allen.

We tried to accommodate the guest star by doing something that he or she was comfortable with. When Michael Redgrave was the guest star, we did a takeoff of *Goodbye, Mr. Chips*. We made Melvyn Douglas, a great leading man who played in over eighty movies, into the head of a hospital with me as one of his doctors.

We had performers who were like utility infielders who could sing and act and had great comedic timing. Robert Preston, who later went on to star on Broadway in *The Music Man*, was wonderful. Eddie Albert, who is probably best known from his work on *Green Acres*, was also excellent.

Jackie Cooper is a Hollywood veteran — an actor, director, producer, and a great drummer. He was a child actor in *The Champ*, *Treasure Island*, and was also one of the Little Rascals. He was very smart and very professional. When he was a guest star, he played in a sketch where I get two tickets to a show — front row seats to the biggest hit in town. Immy and I get to the theater and we come in and sit down. Jackie plays the drummer who starts setting up all this equipment right in front of us with the cymbals right near my head. He builds a monstrosity that almost obstructs our view of the show. When he starts to warm up we ask him, "Are you the drummer?" "No," he says, "I'm just here with the orchestra." Immy and I were sitting there right over the cymbals, and every time he hit them our heads would vibrate.

Rex Harrison was also an excellent guest star. He was both a great comedian and a great actor. He had his own style, very light and gentlemanly. We did a funny sketch together about clothing salesmen. In the first part, I was a customer and he was an American clothier who ran one of those schlock stores you would see on the

Lower East Side of Manhattan, where the guy grabs you and pulls you in, insisting, "Boy, have I got a suit for you. I'll make you this, I'll make you that. You want pleats in the back, I can give you pleats in the back." He played it straight and got a lot of laughs.

For the second part of the sketch, we switched roles and stores. Now the setting is an English men's clothing store. Very chic, very high style. He is now the customer and I am the salesman. The premise is that I won't sell him anything. He walks in and says I'd like to buy a tie. And I say that tie you're wearing is beautiful — you don't need a tie. And he says maybe I should buy a suit? No, no, no. The suit you have on fits you beautifully and will last another hundred years. Well how about a shirt? Oh no, you don't need a shirt.

Finally he says, "How about a collar button?"

And I say, "Would you like gold or ivory?"

"Ivory," he says.

I pick up the phone and say, "Hello, Tanganyika? We have an order for one ivory collar button. Oh, is that right?" I turn back to him and say, "It's too late to shoot an elephant."

Lena Horne was, and still is, a beautiful

woman with a great sense of humor. We gave her a big number where she sang and she was backed up by everybody. Her husband, Lennie Hayton, who was a composer and a musical director, was there and he played for her and orchestrated her music. Today Lena could be part of any sketch, but in those days we couldn't do it. The times would not allow us to put her in a sketch. We couldn't bring on another person of color to play her husband. We couldn't make her somebody's girlfriend or somebody's wife, and we couldn't make her a maid. It would have been too forced. It was all too complicated and too touchy. And it hurt me because I admired her and liked her, and I really wanted to work with her in a sketch.

We also had a problem with the Camel Cigarette Company, which sponsored the first half hour of the show. They refused to allow any performers of color on the air during their slots. Max stood his ground and said, "Now, they will go on in the first act. Let them sing, let them make a living."

We all stood behind Max. The Camel people gave in because they wanted that half hour slot. We chose our moments in those kinds of battles. We weren't trying to rub anyone's nose in anything, but we wanted to make sure that performers got exposure and a check at the end of the week. We had similar fights with the sponsors to have our regulars, the Billy Williams Quartet, be part of the show.

Rudy Vallee had to be the cheapest man in the world. We always tried to be friendly and ask him to come out with us for lunch, and he always politely declined. Later we would always see him in a corner of the same restaurant, eating a sandwich alone. He was afraid he would be stuck picking up someone else's check for $1.20. Because those were the days when a sandwich was eighty cents, celery tonic was ten cents, and a baked apple was fifteen or twenty cents. But we didn't touch Rudy's spending habits on the air. It wasn't our style.

When Jayne Meadows was a guest, we used her in one of our domestic sketches. Immy and I were living in one of those small, middle-class apartments. There's a knock on the door, and Jayne comes in all dolled up and says, "I'm your new neighbor, and I'm having a little cocktail party. I thought maybe the two of you could join me."

I take one look at her and I can't stop saying "Oh boy!" I can't take my eyes off her. She comes by later and asks for some help — she thinks maybe a fuse blew in her apartment. I literally jump up to help. The bit was that I came in with wrenches and more and more tools, humming and singing all the time, and dancing out the door, saying "she needs to have the sinks straightened."

All this is making Immy crazy. "How about our sink?" she yells after me. "Later dear," I yell back. When I suggest that maybe Jayne would like some music and start carrying records over, Immy loses it. She begins breaking the records over my head. "You want more music?" she says. "Here's a waltz!" smashing a record over my head. "Why don't you play this for her while you're in there fixing her apartment," she says. "Here's a foxtrot," smashing another record over my head, "and why don't you play this one, too," followed by another smash.

Someone who was never a credited guest but appeared on *Your Show of Shows* to promote one of his specials was Milton Berle. He asked to use my dressing room, and he was the only guest who ever did.

When we came off a good show where everything worked, including the comedy, the props, the costumes, I would walk away on cloud nine, with a feeling of euphoria that was unparalleled. I felt physically and emotionally strong: I had accomplished something. That feeling would generally last for an hour and a half, which would be followed by the dawning of the realization that it had to be done all over again, the following week, from the beginning.

We only had one day off a week, Sunday, and there were only thirty-five hours between the final curtain and the start of a new show. When I woke up on Sunday morning, the first thing I did was turn on the shower and let it run over me, just to reenter the world. Then I'd start replaying the previous night's show in my head and get apprehensive about the following week, having to do it all over again starting the next morning. If the show was less than spectacular, there was anxiety over making sure next week's show went well. If the show was great, there was anxiety over keeping the streak going.

Often we got into a rhythm. We'd do a good show one week, then a better show the next week, and then an even better one the following week. And then bang! We'd have a week where a couple of sketches were good but the rest of the show was weak. Maybe we had to have that letdown psychologically. It made everyone work harder for the next week.

Not everything worked. But you have to swing hard if you want to hit the home runs. We were giving it our all and we took every loss to heart. My brother Dave would call me and say, "Sid, that one was just for practice. You'll get 'em next week." No one ever bats a thousand or should expect to, and that's probably the most important lesson you can learn in comedy and in life. But when we hit the high notes, glasses shattered all over the country.

During the third and fourth seasons, the weekly grind started to really wear me down. I told Max, "I need a break. I'm starting to meet myself coming in. I'm starting to laugh at the bad jokes." So for two weeks during each of those seasons, Fred Allen guest hosted and did a wonderful job.

Fred Allen was a comic genius. He wrote his own material, including "The Mighty Allen Art Players," which Johnny Carson borrowed from, and was also famous for the long-running radio feud he had with Jack Benny. He was one of the greatest comedy writers and performers in history. I had and still have tremendous respect for him.

As *Your Show of Shows* progressed and gained popularity and prominence, the competition between the comedy sketches and the musical numbers became a great source of frustration for Max and me, as well as the other writers.

The balance between the music and the comedy was initially very successful, particularly for me. Max knew talent when he saw it and didn't hesitate to go after it. He also had a lot of class and style, and the class that he infused into the musical numbers initially lent comparative class and support to the type of comedy I was trying to do. It complemented our style and allowed us to grow and develop the comedy in a refined, creatively charged environment.

Max knew I was a good comedian, but he was very surprised that I knew what I wanted out of the script and the writers. He was out of the Writers' Room after a few months. He trusted us. He was also becoming obsessed with grander and more effusive musical numbers. Very soon after that, he spent more time developing the production numbers with Freddy Fox and less time writing comedy. Often, the last half hour of the show was reserved for light operettas.

Max had veto power, which he used exclusively to cut the comedy. I would tell him, "Max, take out a couple of choruses, they won't miss it." "It's all rehearsed," was his reply. "Take out a couple of lines from the sketches."

The cuts would always have to be made at the last minute, on Saturday evening after the dress rehearsal. I would get the writers together, and it was painful. To get a minute and twenty seconds out of a sketch, you had to cut out a section, not just a line. So we would compromise. We generally looked for the weakest sketch and cut from there, but nobody liked the process. I could never take comedy skits past five or six minutes, eight minutes at the most, because of Max's preference for musical numbers.

Max's vision propelled both him and me to the top. Max thought that the musical numbers were driving the show, but it was a case of the musical tail that was wagging the comedy dog. People were tuning in to see the comedy much more than the elaborate musical numbers. More people wanted to laugh than wanted to hear fifteen choruses of an operetta or a classic aria. They still do. Max had a grand vision. He needed to work with Jeanette MacDonald and

Nelson Eddy in lavish productions of *The Student Prince*. Later on, he would spend a fortune importing ten tons of sand for a desert sketch, where a desert backdrop would have been more than sufficient. But because of his standards he couldn't do things any other way.

We never thought about ending *Your Show of Shows*. As we approached the end of the 1953–1954 season, we thought we would be on NBC for the next ten years. But the networks never tell you what is going to happen. You wake up one morning and read all about it in the newspapers. As *Your Show of Shows* got even more popular with the passage of time, and Max's, Imogene's, and my individual popularity grew, NBC thought it could multiply the benefits and the financial rewards of *Your Show of Shows* by breaking it up into three separate programs. What they didn't want to realize is that they already had three shows: two half hours of comedy and one of music.

NBC executive Hal Janis, a line producer who spoke the network's language, was NBC's permanent liaison to the show. He was a sweet and always mournful looking man, who eventually worried himself to death.

When Hal showed up at my dressing room after all these stories, the first thing I asked was, "What about the rumors?"

"They're true," he said. "There's going to be a shakeup."

"What kind of shakeup?"

"They're going to split you into three parts. Next season, you and Imogene will each get your own shows. Max will get the opportunities to produce his 'spectaculars.' We're going to give him the biggest soundstage in Brooklyn and turn him loose to do all these production numbers he loves so much."

"Why would they want to break up a winning team?" I asked.

"TV is like betting on the horses. And just like the racetrack, three winning combinations are better than one."

I was against breaking up the team, but NBC thought they could cut the baby up. I wanted the opportunity to do bigger sketches. The initial thought was that Imogene would go with me and that Max would go off and produce his musicals. But Imogene's agent was pushing her to go out on her own. NBC gave Max the opportunity to produce one of the first specials, or spectaculars, on television.

On June 5, 1954, after almost 160

episodes, *Your Show of Shows* ended. If you ever get the chance to watch the last program again, you won't be able to miss the emotion of the principals and the company. "It's been a wonderful five years," I told the audience at the curtain. I turned to Imogene. "I just want to say, I love you," and I kissed my tearful colleague.

"We'd like to thank the wonderful audience that we've had," Imogene said. "The audience that's been really terrific to us for all these years, and how grateful all of us are. God bless you."

I then introduced Pat Weaver, who was now the president of NBC. In a very unusual move, he came out, thanked us, and made a short speech about the upcoming season: "Sid, Imogene," he said. "We want to thank you, all of you, all of us at NBC, on or off the *Show of Shows*, all of our advertisers and our viewers for the really spectacular achievement that *Your Show of Shows* has been. And also to tell our viewers about the great plans for all of you for next fall. A new show for Imogene, on Saturday nights at nine o'clock, eastern standard time, every week. And with Sid, a wonderful new hour show on Monday from eight to nine, after the newsreel, eastern standard time. And with Max, a great new special program in color, an hour and a half, on Saturdays and Sundays once a month. Good luck to all of you and these wonderful innovations."

People were very emotional over the end of *Your Show of Shows*. Thousands of letters came in from people who felt like they were losing family. Letting people into their living rooms through the little black-and-white window and getting close to them was a new phenomenon. Saturday nights were about families connecting not only with us but with each other. There was understandable sadness.

Mike Todd, the film producer, was a true showman. He was a Barnum and a Bailey all in one. He was so taken aback when *Your Show of Shows* was canceled that he rented a stadium to honor me. He gave out little cigarette lighters decorated with my picture as a promotion to everyone who came. He had the lights dimmed and everyone in the stadium lit the lighters in tribute. That's what I call a send-off.

As they say in sports, 1954 was a rebuilding year for me. I began putting together my new show, which was to be called *Caesar's Hour*. Without Max and Immy, there was a big void in the production. Every physical aspect of the show changed:

time slot, cast, crew, and writers. The only thing that didn't change one bit was the commitment to deliver first-rate comedy.

When people think about my run on television in the 1950s, they generally don't distinguish between *Your Show of Shows* and *Caesar's Hour*, and I've always taken that as a big compliment. There was a lot of pressure on me to retain the audience and maintain the same level of quality that we'd had for the last four years. After four years of training and learning, I bore ultimate responsibility for *Caesar's Hour*, both in front of and behind the camera.

On *Caesar's Hour*, I was more than just the star; I was now in charge of all aspects of production. The ultimate creative and technical responsibilities — not to mention the challenge to be innovative — rested squarely on my shoulders. There was no more veto power — I was Vito, I was the godfather of the show. I began to grow and the cast, crew, and writers grew along with me.

NBC had used *Your Show of Shows* to successfully develop and capture the Saturday night audience. We had done better than anyone expected against the siren song of Saturday nights out: movies, theater, and the age-old desire to get out of the house.

Staying home and watching television was now an accepted alternative to going out.

Still, it was a great advantage to move to Monday night, traditionally a stay-at-home night for viewers. Sunday night television featured Jack Benny and Ed Sullivan. Tuesday was *I Love Lucy*. Monday was a strong option, even with competition like CBS's *Burns and Allen Show* and *Arthur Godfrey's Talent Scouts*. NBC now had its eye on capturing Monday night, and *Caesar's Hour* was the network's prime-time stalking horse.

The first thing we did was hire a new producer. The William Morris Agency introduced me to Leo Morgan, who was an excellent line producer. He understood the management of a show, from props to scenery. We also got a couple of good directors, including Clark Jones and Frank Bunetta. The assistant director was a man named Heino Ripp, who was able to anticipate and direct the camera shots on the machine because he understood the comedy. He was indispensable to the directors.

Another major advance for the new show was getting the Century Theater, which was on 59th Street and Seventh Avenue. The first thing we did when we got there was clean out the orchestra. We removed every last one of the four hundred seats from that section, which allowed us to shoot a full 360 degrees. The network executives, of course, went nuts: "What the hell are you doing, you're taking away seats." "There are still over nine hundred seats in the loge and balcony," I confidently told them. "That's more than enough for laughs."

Opening up the floor allowed us to create a smaller version of a Hollywood soundstage, with different sets next to each other, which made the live sketches even more realistic. If we were going to do movie satires, it made sense to have the ability to be able to walk from one set to another. We had cameras set up on the stage, in the orchestra section, and in the lobby of the theater. There was a cable man behind each cameraman. It was like a ballet: They had to stay out of each other's way and out of each other's shots. I had a big screen put up over top of the stage, replacing the small monitors that were in awkward locations on either side of the theater so the audience could see the show that was going out over the air to the television audience. The audience initially looked at the stage to see what was going on. Then when the sketches began, they all focused on the big screen. They were able to see close-ups and small gestures clearly. And they all laughed together. At the Center Theater, our previous home, we never used the hydraulics. At the Century Theater, we used everything. It was our collective theatrical training — you use everything you can. And anything we didn't have, we made.

By this time, we also knew much more about the technical and creative process. We were able to build at least two sets at the same time and shoot off of both. When we were on the second stage, we could rebuild the first one so we could generate seamless continuity on a live broadcast.

While the sketches for *Your Show of Shows* ran for five to six minutes, those on *Caesar's Hour* went up to twenty minutes and longer. The sketches were not only longer, they were more sophisticated, and they reflected four years' worth of growth and maturity. Max and I were no longer bucking up against each other over cuts of what seemed like an ever-growing number of encores.

Part of the romance and the beauty of early television was that you knew everyone, including the crew. There was less distance and more communication than there is now on these types of shows. Everyone felt part of a family. A lot of people got their start on our show, including Hugh Downs, who was an announcer and later went on to a distinguished career as a television journalist and Don Pardo, who later became the announcer on *Jeopardy!* and *Saturday Night Live*.

We got a great break when we got the *Your Show of Shows* camera crew for *Caesar's Hour*. They were the best NBC had, and, like a sports franchise, they traveled as a team. There was a level of excellence that permeated everywhere, a collective willingness to go the extra mile. The soundman wouldn't come in with two or three potential effects, he'd bring in between ten and fifteen. The costume designers were meticulous and creative about the preparation of the costumes. There was a tremendous sense of excitement and pride at being associated with the show.

Carl, Howie, and I had just come off our best season of *Your Show of Shows*, which included the classic "This Is Your Story" parody. We were at the top of our game. The three of us had years of experience under our belts, we knew each other's moves and rhythms. Plus we had the confidence, the ability, and the resources to experiment with our craft and take risks even in the live format. We used each other as a means to propel ourselves higher creatively, but also as a safety net to protect each other from the inevitable mistakes of the live format.

Carl would often bring his young son, Rob, to watch the show. Rob Reiner learned at a young age about storytelling with a beginning, a middle, and an end and he learned early how to keep an audience's interest. Now, as a filmmaker, he's got a body of excellent work to prove it.

I would often open the show with a greeting and some kind of summary that gave the audience an idea of what was in store for them. I generally wore a robe with a costume on underneath: I had to be ready for the sketch that would commence seconds after the introduction. I always closed with a variation of "Thank you, good night, and God bless you." Even though I didn't have a signature sign on or sign off, the closest I ever came is the way I've signed autographs for the last thirty years: "With love and laughter." I have always believed that if you have both love and laughter in your life, you have it all.

Since I was now a businessman as well as a performer, I formed a production company, called Shelric after my daughter

Michele, whom we called Shelly, and my son, Rick. When my daughter Karen was born in 1956, we added a *k* to the end of the company name. We took office space on the top two floors of the Milgram Building on Fifth Avenue and 57th Street, across the street from Tiffany's. I had a penthouse office with an open-air terrace. There was a large teakwood desk with canvasses by Rouault and Cezanne on the walls. When things got too hectic, I used to go up there and just sit and listen to Beethoven or Rachmaninoff. It was as special as it sounds.

We custom built our office space, so we could rehearse the sketches on the top floor and the dance numbers on a lower floor. Everything was done simultaneously because there was still less than a week to prepare for the live show.

The budget for the show was now at $125,000 a week, which may seem like peanuts when you compare it to the fact that today some shows pay millions of dollars an episode just in salaries. But it was a significant increase over the budget for *Your Show of Shows*, which was $64,000 per episode, as well as the comparatively meager $19,000 a week we had to play with on the *Admiral Broadway Revue*.

We were spending money, but we were delivering quality merchandise. *Caesar's Hour* sketches had elaborate sets, while most of the sketches on *Your Show of Shows* had the scenery painted against the wall, with just a table and chairs on the stage. I even had input into the construction of the sets, which was not always a good thing. One week in frustration over not getting a scene right, I punched a set and put a hole in it. After that, they built sets that they could turn around so that they could hide any holes I happened to punch in them.

Caesar's Hour premiered on Monday, September 27, 1954. Our first guest was the Italian star Gina Lollobrigida, who was known as "the most beautiful woman in the world," "the Mona Lisa of the twentieth century," and "the best thing to come out of Italy since spaghetti." It was going to be her first time acting on American television.

We had initially thought of a sketch with Gina as an earthy peasant woman working in the fields, but we realized that she would probably want to look glamorous in front of 60 million people. So we came up with a sketch about a contest, and the guy that wins the contest gets to go out on a date with Gina Lollobrigida.

She was a lovely woman. Her husband, a doctor, would not allow her to be alone with any man. And she knew where the camera was — we had to build a special staircase so she could make a grand entrance. But all she worried about was how her dress fit. It was always "a little longer in the back, a little tighter in the front." "Gina," I kept saying, "we have to rehearse the sketch." "You'll see the dress," was her reply, "and that will be that." She wouldn't leave the dressing room; she kept being refitted. This was my opening show, I thought, and I'm worried about a staircase and a tight dress. Something must be wrong.

Gina worked out fine but after the second show, we realized that we needed a woman, or, more specifically, a female lead. While we never thought of Imogene as replaceable by anyone, we knew that we needed a regular female character to complete the ensemble.

I started looking around, preferably for someone I'd worked with before. Nanette Fabray had been a guest on *Your Show of Shows*, where she had been very good in a silent movie sketch. I had also met her a few years earlier. When I was doing *Make Mine Manhattan*, she was at the theater next door doing *High Button Shoes*.

Nanette was a different type of performer. She was what the French call a soubrette: she could sing, dance, act, and look beautiful. She had perfect timing and a sense of comedy and I knew she had scope. But when I put a call in to her, she told me she had just come out of the hospital.

A few months earlier, Nanette had been told that she was going to lose her hearing, a nightmare for an actor. That never happened, but the prognosis understandably caused her to have a breakdown and landed her in a hospital for a few months.

Nanette told me about what had befallen her and said she wasn't sure that she could handle a weekly show. "I can't remember lines," she said. "I can't do this, I can't do that." I wasn't fazed. I told her she was coming to work with us. "Don't worry," I said. "We'll help you." She looked good and she felt good, and she had the experience of Broadway. What more did you need?

You can't compare Nanette and Imogene other than that they were both amazingly talented performers. Their theatrical training was immensely helpful to both of them in their work on live television, which was essentially a filmed theatrical performance. They each brought different skills and strengths to the stage. Like Imogene,

Nanette covered me in takes and was also able to find her own takes. A wonderful singer, Nanette also did musical numbers on her own.

Sadly, Nanette left after our second season because of contract disputes. Her agent told her that she was getting laughs by herself and should have her own show. He made such large demands, we couldn't meet them. Even if we could, the rapport between us probably would not have been the same.

During our last season, we had Janet Blair in that role. Janet, as I mentioned, had been the lead in the film version of *Tars and Spars*. She had good comic timing but was not a comedienne nearly at the level of Imogene or Nanette. It didn't work. There was no chemistry between us. It was very frustrating.

Caesar's Hour went off the air in May 1957, after three seasons. There was no one reason but a number of them, each true to varying degrees, why the show was losing its steam and slipping in the ratings. For one thing, as the television audience was expanding outside of the big cities, audience tastes were changing and attention spans were shrinking. They didn't understand the foreign movies we were parodying.

We were writing high-class comedy and were not willing to dumb it down.

But that wasn't the only reason we lost the ratings. During the third year of *Caesar's Hour*, the network wanted to capitalize on the success of our time slot, so they started using us as a stalking horse to launch other shows. We would be on for three weeks, and then the fourth week would be used to feature a special by Jimmy Durante or Martin and Lewis. You always need to manage the audience's expectations. Once you break the cycle, it's over.

NBC then moved us back to Saturday night, where we competed against the immensely popular Lawrence Welk. Singers of all kinds started climbing the TV charts: not only Lawrence Welk but Perry Como, Andy Williams, and Dean Martin. Singers supplanted revue comedies, and comedians no longer dominated the airwaves. It was the end of an era for comedians, and the variety show never really made a comeback. With the exception of the *Carol Burnett Show*, the *Sonny and Cher Show*, and the *Flip Wilson Show*, there was nothing in the prime-time variety format that held the attention of the public for very long.

Personally, I reacted to the ratings drop

badly. I became angry and self-critical. It became an almost self-fulfilling prophecy as I watched my timing slip. I had been on for nine straight years, I was bushed, I'd had enough. The network knew that I was drinking heavily and that I was collapsing under the pressure of weekly live television. It wasn't publicly known, but the network knew. Yet no one came to me as they did to Kelsey Grammar and many others years later and said, "Sid, look what you're doing to yourself. Why don't you take time off and go somewhere where you can relax and get better. Go rest and then you can come back to work." When you're on that kind of merry-go-round, somebody has to help you get off.

Even if they had a show that was successful in the ratings and making money, the network never took care of its people. NBC had the rebel debel army mentality about its celebrities: if they don't fit, we'll get another one. As comedians fell in battle or ratings, they could be replaced. The whole industry took the position that talent was fungible. The feeling was that you could get great comedians by the dozen, simply by shaking a tree. Network executives really had the mindset that they could stick their heads out their doors and say: "Get me another Chaplin or W. C. Fields," and that they could be pulled off the corner where they were hanging around. After a while they found out that without the right performer, the show didn't go that well. They had the same writers, the same words being written, but it wasn't as funny.

Every comedian that NBC had was ultimately brought over by William Paley at CBS, who stole every major talent from NBC over the next few years: Jimmy Durante, Groucho Marx, Burns and Allen, Jack Benny, myself. NBC fired Pat Weaver at the same time we left the air. After that, NBC didn't have one show in the top ten for a few years.

After *Caesar's Hour* ended, I did an awful lot of specials that were sponsored by Chevrolet and written by Larry Gelbart and Woody Allen. I worked with real pros like Art Carney, José Ferrer, Audrey Meadows, Shirley MacLaine, and Paul Douglas. Paul was not only a lovely man but also a wonderful comedic actor. In one sketch, he plays a financially successful man who shares the secret of his success with me over dinner: "I'm a successful guy, because I don't use cash. I owe everyone. I'm in debt for over $150,000. I don't pay for anything!"

I played a man who was getting married at a large group wedding. When the minister finishes the ceremony, I am married to the woman who is standing on the other side of me, instead of my fiancée. I start complaining to the minister, who says, "I always marry to the right."

"I married the wrong woman!"

"People marry the wrong people every day," he replies.

I look at my fiancée and feel sorry for her. I then look at the other woman, the one that I was married to. She is beautiful. I start thinking, and then I smile and turn back to my exasperated fiancée. "I will straighten this out. I promise . . . I'll call you next week. Thursday. Friday, the latest."

In another sketch, Paul Douglas and I play scientists who send a termite into space to expose it to cosmic rays. As we retrieve the capsule, while I reach in to get the termite, it bites my finger. Moments later I develop an insatiable appetite for wood, ripping the arm off a chair and eating it. Audrey plays my wife. I get home just in time to celebrate my wooden anniversary, and what I do to celebrate is eat the chair, the floor, and the piano. It was a fun sketch that was based on all the B movie science fiction thrillers of the 1940s and 1950s.

Two short years later, a young man named Stan Lee wrote a comic book about a teenager who gets bitten by a radioactive spider and develops remarkable powers. I assume Stan Lee was a fan of our shows. Although I can't prove it, I suspect Larry Gelbart and Woody Allen may be indirectly responsible for the creation of Spider-Man.

We created magic with the new medium of live television. For almost nine years, people rushed home early on Saturday nights, or if they didn't have a television set of their own, ran to their neighbors to watch us. Our work has been credited for setting the stage, figuratively and literally, for almost every variety show and sketch and parody-driven program from *Saturday Night Live* to *Monty Python's Flying Circus*. We made the rules, broke new ground, and had a lot of fun and interesting times.

Our early successes helped television attain the level of success and importance that it has today. TV is the most important thing we have now. It is the primary source for news and entertainment all over the world. Everything is brought to your home through television. It's the great equalizer and a big part of democracy. You can see almost anything you want, and you get to make up your own mind.

Though only a fraction of today's audience is old enough to have seen me in my prime, more than half a century later, people still come up to me and thank me for the wonderful laughter and seeing their parents laughing. I am grateful and proud of the accomplishment.

Chapter 7

THE WRITERS' ROOM

For nine years, I presided over what was arguably the best collection of comedy writers ever assembled in the history of television, and possibly in the history of the written word — unless you think the U.S. Constitution is funny.

Think of the chariot race in *Ben-Hur*. That's what it felt like — as if I had a team of magnificent horses that could take me anywhere I wanted to go, and fast. I felt like Francis X. Bushman or Charlton Heston driving those chariots in the Circus Maximus. Anything I asked of the team, they gave. That to me was the thrill of a life-time, to sit there and throw out ideas. Any idea I came up with would be fleshed out by brilliant people who knew what they were doing, and they were funny. Maybe the most important thing I did on the show was to sit with and preside over that group of geniuses. There are probably few shows in television history where the producers, performers, and writers were so attuned to each other's talents and strengths as we were then. And we are the only show in history where the writers became as famous as the performers.

I called the Writers' Room the sanctum sanctorum. If you look those words up you'll see they come from the biblical phrase "holy of holies," which is an indication of how important I thought the place was. The show began in that room, where young, creative people were pitching ideas, catching them in the air, and putting them down on the written page. If it's not on the page, it's not on the stage. As Neil Simon would later write, one of my greatest gifts was that I understood the connection between the page and the stage.

Every morning, I would walk into the room, sit down in my chair, and shoot the breeze for a few minutes with the writers. I then lit a cigar, which was the signal to start working, and said: "All right, let's hear the brilliance." It was hilarious torture. I was tough and demanding, but I think I was fair, and to a certain degree, nurturing. I demanded the best from my writers and I always got it. They each knew what we were working for. Good was never good enough.

Lucille Kallen once joked that "Sid is the

only man with 32,000 writers, each of whom is solely responsible for his success." It's a funny line, and in a way, it's very true. I am grateful to each one of my writers for their respective contribution to my success.

Every artist creates in his or her own way. When Michelangelo went to Rome and saw the statues, I can imagine him saying, how can I be different, how can I top this? And he sculpted Moses. Because of the cut of the marble, he had to settle for a sitting Moses. But he put one foot forward, making Moses looking like he was going to rise. When you look at his Moses, you can see beyond the actual physical statue, you can see the artist. One of the things that I am most proud of in my career is that every writer that left the show, without exception, went on to do great, landmark, classic work, that both entertained and inspired others after them. That's a legacy I am especially proud of.

The experience of the Writers' Room was quintessentially American — talented, industrious people coming together to create. Good people don't mind working together. They just want to be appreciated and treated fairly. I made sure journalists spoke to the writers for interviews as well as the stars of the program. The writers helped each other every day and I helped them believe in themselves.

The writers were in effect my Praetorian Guard. We were the New York Yankees and the Duke Ellington Band. After a few years, we were all seasoned. There may not have been consistent affection, but there was mutual respect, creative competition, and what is now called synergy. Each writer had his own style and virtually created schools of comedy. They each contributed to the room individually, but more importantly they were able to write together as a team. Once Larry Gelbart was asked why all of my writers tended to be young and Jewish. "Probably because all of our parents were old and Jewish," was his reply.

The Writers' Room was immortalized on television in the classic *Dick Van Dyke Show*, which Carl Reiner created and wrote; in the charming film *My Favorite Year*, which Mel Brooks created and produced; and in Neil Simon's hilarious play *Laughter on the 23rd Floor*. People have always tried to replicate the magic of the Writers' Room, not only in the entertainment arena but also in many other creative environments. To this day, shows use the title "head writer" with the highest respect and as a tribute to the prototype we created in the '50s.

There was also a mystique about the show at NBC while it was being done. The executives did not believe it. "We're getting an hour and a half show every week and it's good — how do you do it?" And the response was always: "Don't ask questions you don't want to hear the answers to. Never look a gift horse in the mouth."

People always ask me whether the crazy stories you hear about that room were true. Since I was there, I am in a position to know the answer: Many of them were and some of them weren't. Certainly the spirit was there. The energy that existed inside the walls of the Writers' Room as we created was palpable. We laughed a lot, we screamed a lot, and then we hollered a lot. It was a combination of euphoria and terror.

The energy in the Writers' Room was like a cyclotron — someone would come up with an idea and it would stimulate another idea and we would build on it. No one ever finished a sentence that I can remember. There was a healthy competition, like a bunch of pups in a big litter. You got mad for a couple of seconds, laughed for a few more seconds, and then you moved on. Anger built up like thunder and lightning, you heard the crash, and then it was over.

Samuel Goldwyn once said, "From a

polite conference comes a polite script." That is the way I felt about the Writers' Room. There had to be fire in the room in order for there to be fire in the sketch. There was never politeness, but there was always creativity, respect, and product. In the Writers' Room, if you could hear yourself, nothing was happening.

But if it was a free-for-all, it was a free-for-all with order. Like the chaos theory in physics. The best finally gets through — it was based strictly on that. No one person wrote anything and nobody wrote alone. It was group writing at its finest: everything was agreed on by the group. Unless there was a song, which Mel Tolkin and Shelley Keller would go off and write in ten minutes, we all wrote together.

The writers needed to show that they were their own people. And they were all proud of their ideas and their work. They didn't have to be afraid of anybody. They each could have gotten writing jobs anywhere, but they liked the action and the atmosphere in that room.

In the Writers' Room, we relied not on jokes per se but on characterization. I would throw out jokes that were funny but had nothing to do with the sketch and would hold it up and break the rhythm.

After we got the laugh, we had to take it back in. A joke, even if it was funny, could send the sketch in the wrong direction. The jokes had to grow out of the situation. Each of us would try to make the sketches as good and as funny as they could be. Each writer contributed in a different fashion and we all complemented each other. The magic was in those collaborative skills. Carl Reiner could find great pieces of business. Larry Gelbart was a great dialogue man. Neil Simon was a great storyteller. Mel Brooks, God bless him, could always come up with some hysterical shtick.

If you wanted to put it into musical terms, you'd say the Writers' Room functioned like an orchestra. Each writer was a different instrument, using different timbres and harmonies. You want a piccolo and a bass. Mel Tolkin kept the rhythm — he was a superb structure guy. And Mel Brooks was the cymbals — he didn't keep the rhythm, and he always went for the biggest bang he could get away with.

Another thing. When you came into the Writers' Room, you checked your ego at the door. In the room I was no big shot. There were no big shots. The big shot of the moment was the person who came up with the most recent funny situation, line, or bit. He or she could strut around while the other writers were seething and creatively scrambling for their next moment in the sun.

The Writers' Room was more than just a place; it was a state of mind and a standard to aspire to. Part of the mystique and the appeal of the space, not only for people in show business but for people from every profession and walk of life, stems from the fact that amid all the frenetic energy, the yelling, and the chaos, these were all people who loved coming to work every day. They were people who thoroughly enjoyed what they were doing. How many individuals can say that they love their work, or respect the people that they work with, or talk about it with such fond recollections more than fifty years later?

That euphoria manifested itself in countless situations where I would walk into that room with an idea for the following week, have the confidence that it could be fleshed out and developed, then watch the idea evolve from the writers' often initially incredulous reaction to a full-blown sketch.

With the exception of Max, who was in his late forties, we were a very young group charged with the responsibility of creating the equivalent of a full-scale Broadway show every week. When *Your Show of Shows* started, I was twenty-seven, just turning twenty-eight. The other writers were about my age, except for Mel Brooks, who was only twenty-three. We were young men and women just pushing the envelope, saying, "let's do it." Week after week, we were together. We were like a family that relied on each other.

When Orson Welles made *Citizen Kane*, he brought his troupe of young actors from the Mercury Theater in New York City out to Hollywood. He wanted stage actors who had never been in a film before because he did not want them to be held back by the knowledge of what they could not do. He wanted people who could do scenes in one take. Similarly, we had the license to do it and we didn't have the insecurity of knowing that it couldn't be done.

I often think that the most important aspect of this working environment was that when we went out to lunch, we all sat at the same table and we all laughed together. We would also socialize together outside of work. I respected all of my writers and worked hard to maintain their respect. We were all in the same boat. Or, if you prefer military metaphors, we were all in the trenches together. It was like being in a war, being a soldier next to other soldiers in a foxhole under fire where all of a sudden these guys become your buddies.

My management style was to be part of the process from the moment of inception. We wrote together, page by page, note by note. The way you manage is by doing. You have to show people what you want. Talk it over. Just don't say, "Hey, let's do a sketch about this." Every show has a different way of working. My way of working was to sit in the room together, from the page one/scene one "Hello dear, I'm home," all the way to the punch line. I contributed. They contributed more than I did — but I would try it on for them. I had to feel good about each sketch because I was the one who had to perform it. If an idea didn't fit right, we'd redo it. That's why it didn't feel so bad if I had to shoot an idea down.

Other stars of variety shows would have the script sent upstairs and slipped under the door. They'd read it and make marks on it and send it back down for rewrites. I thought that was the biggest waste of time. I preferred being there when the ideas germinated. I could try something on for size; see if an idea had legs. If they started to come up with something and I didn't even like the idea, if I was in the room, it was gone with the speed of light. You could turn one down right there before any time was spent on it, saving hours and hours. You see how the idea formed and if you didn't like the way it was going, you could change it different ways, and then change it again because you had a clear idea of the context and its genesis. Good ideas became better without hesitation or muddling.

Before *Your Show of Shows* became a hit, we were on a very tight budget and we had the cheapest offices we could rent. The very first Writers' Room was the dressing room in our offices on 56th Street, right near Nola Studios, which was over the original Lindy's Restaurant. During the first year of *Your Show of Shows*, I remember that the room overlooked *Mister Roberts*, the toast of Broadway.

These were the days when old New York buildings were really old New York buildings. The elevators were like steel cages. When you pulled back the gated door, it sprang back like a trap. We were writing amid women's underwear, socks, and jock straps. It wasn't what you'd call conducive to the creative process.

Once *Your Show of Shows* became a hit, we could afford better office space. Max took offices at the City Center and we wrote the show in Max's L-shaped office in

Suite 6-M. The Writers' Room was now fancy enough to have a couch and two chairs. During the early days, Max sat in on the writing sessions from behind his desk. He would contribute to the mix, but as I grew as a comedian and a writer, he became less involved in the comedy aspect of the show.

Max didn't understand a lot of what we wanted to do. His humor was more in the vein of "What if Christopher Columbus was an usher at the Roxy Theater," or "what if Babe Ruth sold hot dogs in the stands at Yankee Stadium?" There was no vision and no range to the comedy. We were writing sketches off sophomoric premises. I hated it and soon enough Max left us alone to create the comedy. What we did was the very beginning of television sketch comedy; it was the cracking of the creative egg. We were just pecking out of the shell. Every Monday morning for thirty-nine weeks a year, we faced the same task: creating six comedy sketches in three days. That was easier said than done. Since these were the days before fancy copying and collating machines, the show had to be written by Wednesday night to allow time for the mimeograph machines to crank out duplicate scripts and for orchestration, props, scenery, costumes, makeup, and sound effects to be readied for

Saturday night's live performance, not to mention the fact that we first had to work on the actual show run-throughs, rewriting, blocking, and rehearsals.

But on Monday morning when we came in we did not have the slightest idea of what we were going to do. All of our energies had been focused on the creation of the prior week's show. We didn't have a chance to think ahead. We christened the beginning of the week "Bloody Monday" because we walked into the room with no material. Everything we had the week before, we'd used up. It was the fear that all writers face: the crisis of the empty page. We had three days to pitch lines and ideas and create six complete sketches, which had to be scripted and put into the hopper.

We had to start somewhere, so we'd talk over what we'd seen on TV the night before, all the big shows that were on Sunday night: Ed Sullivan, Jack Benny, Fred Allen. We would talk about what they did and how they did it and whether it was done well, but we would never get any ideas from them. We would also critique our own work. We never actually watched it because we didn't have time to run the show. About 9:30 I'd light up a cigar and we'd go to work.

There was no playbook, there was no basis

or theme from which we could vary for an hour-and-a-half live show, or how to write for television at all for that matter. Unlike comedy today, which has over five decades of solid reference material, we were mining everything to find new ideas. Ideas came from everywhere and anywhere: our own lives, friends and relatives, movies and music. We were making it up as we were going along.

Sitting in a room where time was easily measured by the accumulation of dozens of empty coffee cups and hundreds of cigar and cigarette butts, we would crank out scripts. *Your Show of Shows* and *Caesar's Hour* for me were graduate school after the colleges of the Catskills, the Coast Guard, and Hollywood. It was almost like an academic research project because we tried things that were out there that had never been done before. And we were all learning and growing together.

We looked for ideas anywhere we could find them. We came up with a character called "The Mumbler," based on a man I ran into in Manhattan. I was in a Chock Full o' Nuts one day, and there was a man sitting next to me who was talking out loud to himself while he was eating. He was arguing with himself: "It's raining on my day off." He was mad because it was his day off and it was spoiled because it was raining. He was totally out of it.

Out of curiosity, I followed him for about twelve blocks. He changed his mind ten times. "Look at the pigeons. Maybe I'll go to the zoo." He got on a bus and a little old lady came on and he started to mumble. He said, "Nobody's gonna give you a seat. She'll stay there till she'll collapse. See that, she collapsed! That's the way the world is, lady. You're gonna lay there. You're gonna stay there on the floor. Nobody's gonna pick you up!" And that was a sketch.

Because we didn't have time for an outside life, we were especially desperate for ideas. We'd all be asking each other, "Did anybody go anywhere? Did anybody do anything? Does anybody know anybody who did anything?" One Monday we had nothing to write; we were blank. Somebody said, "I just moved into a new building and the walls are so thin it's ridiculous. I mean I saw the blue light of the television in the next apartment coming through the wall." Bang! That was the idea. From that we crafted a sketch about a man in the middle of an apartment house able to see and hear everything that went on in his building. Like the old Tony Martin song, it was part of "The Tenement Symphony."

Because we wrote about the human condition, it was assumed that we had material everywhere. Fred Allen once joked, "Caesar's material is all around him and inexhaustible. Caesar running out of material is like NBC running out of vice presidents." That may have been true, but mining the material for the gold was still an arduous task. And mining, as you know, is a dirty and dangerous business.

The time pressures were so great I took the telephone out of the room. Actually, the phone had rung once during an idea and disrupted the creative flow, and I literally ripped it out of the wall and threw it into the hallway. Other than emergencies, there were no calls during working hours. And I meant it. Because the script had to be finished on Wednesday, sometimes we'd have to compromise because we just couldn't come up with that indescribable "it." So you settled — you had to. Not every sketch was a diamond. Some had a couple of flaws. There was one time when Wednesday night came but we just couldn't get it. We usually turned the script in at 6:00 p.m. but it wasn't finished. "All right," I said, "let's break for dinner. We'll have a nice meal, we'll relax and we'll come back and we'll finish this." So we all had dinner, got back

to the office about 8:00 p.m., and started to write. And boy were we excited about what we were coming up with.

But when we came in the next morning, our reactions were more like we were smelling bad fish. "Who wrote this? This is terrible!" Because we really wanted to get home, unconsciously we were settling for things we normally wouldn't have. And we never did that again.

I also believed that after you eat, you couldn't think or perform that well. You're sluggish. You're not ready to do battle with either the page or the stage. When you get up in the morning, and you've had breakfast, and you've fought traffic to get in, you're mad at this, you're mad at that, you're pumped up and ready to do battle. Which is the way it ought to be.

Thursday was the most creative day of the week. It was also the most stressful day. Nothing was complete yet; everything was "in half." We had the page, now we had to get it to the stage. We all got together in a big rehearsal room and put the whole show up on its feet, taking the ideas and putting meat around them. We found things: pieces of business that related to the sketches, additional dialogue, things that we could do with and to each other. We

could match the business to the dialogue. We knew what to look for. We'd add things to the script, cut things out, and make changes on the spot. The writers were right there, watching and studying.

We were helped by very good directors, including Bill Hobin, who was great at picking shots and ran the show, and Greg Garrison, a very talented and very flamboyant man who later went on to work with Dean Martin. Immy, Carl, Howie, and I would also direct each other in the execution of the sketches. Once we got the words out of the way, we gave the sketches room to breathe. We would wait for each other, and we could time each other, which let us see the idiosyncrasies in the themes and the dialogue.

We were focused on the characters we were playing, but at the same time, loose enough and versatile enough to compensate for the audience responses and for the latitude we needed to give to each other as performers. As soon as we felt comfortable with our lines, sometimes while we were still in the office, we would do a loose blocking. We would rehearse all the places that we'd have to hit onstage. There were black lines, blue lines, red lines, yellow lines, green lines, purple lines, which all corresponded to different scenes where the

scenery had to be put and where the camera had to focus.

While all this was going on, we also had to make sure that we weren't looking down on the floor at the marks. In order to remember all the moves I needed to make and so I could see where I was going, I would associate each move I had made in my mind with a gesture that would fit with what I was doing in the sketch. That would allow me to look for the mark without appearing awkward or conspicuous. I'd fit it into the acting so I would know where I would have to be. We didn't just wait for our cues, we listened to each other. And if you listen, you look like you're listening, and you are able to get your fellow actor's tempo and thrust.

In addition to the marking and the blocking, once we went live we were also mining the audience for any sort of additional laughter. If any of us found a bit that could extend the humor for a few more seconds, we'd do it. That was a laugh over and above what we thought we were going to get. Then we would come back to the script. We looked for that with every show and with every sketch.

By the time we got to the live show on Saturday night, we had gone through four rehearsals. The first time there was a loose blocking, which was followed by a tighter blocking. Friday was a complete run-through without a stop for the technical people. The cameramen studied the shots; the costumes and props were tested and altered as necessary. On Saturday at 10:00 a.m. we'd have a full dress rehearsal during the day, and then we'd go out live at nine o'clock. Even this late, we never thought about the following week's show. We were still writing the current week's installment right up to curtain time. The writers were there, watching, making suggestions, and contributing additional dialogue. They stayed there right through the actual live broadcast, watching from the control room, often making changes through to the time the sketch was performed live. It was an extremely dedicated and passionate group.

Part of the romance and the beauty of early television was that you knew everyone, including the crew. They were all part of the family, excited and proud to work there. The cameramen tried to get the best shots, the set designers and the costumers were always trying to do one better. There was less distance and more communication than there is now on these types of shows. Although even today when there is a hit show, the cast and crew become a family, which is one of the most wonderful aspects of the television business.

The first writers we brought in to write for *Your Show of Shows* were Mel Tolkin and Lucille Kallen, both veterans of the *Admiral Broadway Revue*. Mel Tolkin was with me from day one through the close of *Caesar's Hour* and even beyond that for a few specials. He was a little older than the other writers, more mature, and he really earned the title of head writer. Mel was the whip. He helped manage this creative — and very unmanageable — crew. If I had to be away for a couple of hours for a network meeting or some public relations work, Mel would make sure that the script would get written and exercise as much control as you could over a group of explosively creative writers not known for their decorum.

Mel was part of a tradition of humor stemming from the stark oppression of European Jews, a tradition that could find the funny side of the direst situation, even a pogrom. He could come up with a sketch out of anything. He had and still has a very literate style and a quiet dignity. Mel was not only street smart, he was book smart. Mel was also the foreign influence. He was a Russian immigrant with a thick accent to prove it, and he had a distinctly European perspective. Mel would later go on to write for Danny Kaye and for the landmark *All in the Family*.

Mel Tolkin and Carl Reiner are the strongest arguments I know for artistic talent in the gene pool. Mel's son Michael is an accomplished author and screenwriter. Our kids grew up together. Mel and I still get together for lunch. We have a bond that people can tell exists by just looking at our body language. When we are with a group he always sits next to me, with his quiet loyalty, integrity, and sharp wit.

Lucille was a very smart and very businesslike woman. She provided the woman's point of view, which was crucial. While everyone else was jumping around, yelling and screaming ideas and dialogue, she was the one with the pencil and paper in charge of following my direction, putting things down and ultimately editing it into a working script. Often she would wave her sweater in the air like a flag to get the attention she needed to get a line or an idea in.

When *Your Show of Shows* began, Mel Brooks could be found hanging around the Writers' Room. He was initially an uncredited writer, contributing random jokes and ideas. His name didn't appear as a member of the writing staff on the closing credits, or crawl, at the end of the show until late in the first season. Mel was persistent: He was pushing his way into the Writers' Room, through a combination of raw talent, inertia, and sheer chutzpah. Had today's union rules been in place, Mel couldn't have gotten the entrée he had and advanced the way he did. He instinctively knew what I was trying to do with my comedy, that I was a storyteller interpreting real-life situations, as opposed to a riff comic. I immediately saw Mel's gift of pure, off-the-wall humor and kept him on. He knew how to punch up a scene or give a bit the right spin to make it funny. I offered to pay him $40 a week out of my own pocket. He took the $40 and then later came back to me, telling me he needed more money.

"How much do you need?" I asked him.

"I need at least $50 a week," he said.

"Fifty dollars is unheard of," I told him. "But I will give you $45 if Max will agree to give you the other $5."

Max point-blank refused: "I won't pay $5 for that." So I started Mel out at $40 a week, which was not a bad salary in those days. Rent was $20 a month. If you were making $50 a week, you got married.

Mel told me that he couldn't make ends meet on $40 a week and — to prove this —

took me to where he lived in Greenwich Village. It was a cellar on Broome Street outfitted with a bed, a chair, a toilet, a stove, and an icebox. This wasn't a hovel; he was living underneath a hovel. After one look at the apartment, I raised his salary to $50 a week.

Mel was often the joke machine. You could give him a topic and he could shoot back a joke. If you said carrots, he would say, "There was this guy couldn't get to sleep because he ate too many carrots. Every time he closed his eyes he would see through the lids." Once I took Mel by the head and announced, "This is mine." Without missing a beat, Mel fished my wallet out of my pocket, waved it in the air and said, "This is mine."

Mel was the kind of guy, even walking down the street you never knew what he was going to say. Once he passed two nuns and he cracked, "You're out of the sketch." One of his earliest contributions to the show was an off-the-wall airport interview sketch. I played a Stanislavski disciple, Ivan Ivanovich, who illustrates his version of method acting by imitating a pinball gyrating around the pinball machine.

Max would fire Mel at least once a week. Sometimes once a day. Not that it inhibited Mel. He actually used to taunt Max. When Max would yell at him, "You're nothing, all you'll ever be is nothing," Mel would respond, without missing a beat, "And you're the boss over nothing!"

When Max wasn't in the office, Mel would sit in Max's chair, put his feet up on the desk, and chomp on one of Max's cheap, foul-smelling cigars. He would get up on Max's desk and imitate him. Occasionally Max would walk in and catch Mel *in flagrante impersonato*. One way Max tried to manage Mel's manic enthusiasm was by throwing lit cigars at him. They weren't just lit; Max blew on them to make them hotter. But Max knew what we all knew, that Mel was making a significant contribution to the show. Otherwise he would have only fired Mel once, for real.

The insomniac Mel was also in the habit of coming in late. He was at least an hour behind schedule every day. He would tell me, "Sid, I can't sleep, I just can't get to sleep at night," which was a logic I could never understand. "Well, geez," I'd say, "then why are you so late? If you can't sleep you should be here early." He was full of excuses: "There was a bad light on Sixth Avenue. A window washer got stuck."

The perpetually late Mel would always burst into Max's office and slide across the room like he was going toward second base

(Carl would always yell, "Safe!"), which would be Max's cue to start yelling and throw his cigar at him. Once Mel made his entrance, threw his straw hat across the room and said, "Lindy made it!" We couldn't help laughing, and at that point, yelling at Mel was moot as well as futile. Mel's tardiness was also a function of his not wanting to be involved in the foundation work for the sketches. He wasn't interested in the initial development. He wanted to punch things up.

Mel always phoned ahead to the coffee shop downstairs and ordered a bagel and coffee to precede him. It was his way of announcing that he was on his way. Because he was never there when the bagel and coffee arrived, somebody else would always pay for it. The writers eventually complained about both the bagels and the lateness. "Sid," they said, "you have to do something about it."

The next time the delivery boy showed up with the coffee and bagel, I took care of it. I gave the kid a twenty-dollar bill. Mel sauntered in with his usual "I'm sorry I'm late. Where's my coffee and bagel?" He had the fifty-cent piece in his hand ready to hand to whoever paid for his breakfast.

Handing him the bag, I said, "That'll be $20."

"What do you mean?"

"I paid for your coffee," I said. "And I'm a very big tipper."

"Oh, you didn't have to do that."

I said, "Mel, if you don't want to come on time, it's going to cost you $20 a day. And I may raise it to $50 if I like the delivery guy." Negative cash flow caught Mel's attention. He still wound up coming in late, but not that late. Twenty minutes or a half hour was forgiven.

When Mel would get an idea, he would jump up against the wall or onto the couch and yell, "Listen — I got it! I got it! I got it!" A lot of times he did and a lot of times he didn't and he would slowly creep off the couch. Mel was our off-the-wall guy. He was in charge of delivering the unexpected.

Mel was also relentless in trying to sell an idea. Once he was so excited he followed me down 56th Street trying to convince me to use one. When I continued to decline, he actually poked me in the chest. "Caesar, you do that joke!" he said, poking me again for emphasis. I never liked anyone touching me in the first place. But two fingers in the chest particularly aroused my ire. I didn't know at the time whether to tear him in two, snap him apart, or maybe break him into many pieces. "Mel, did you see what you just did?" "Yes," he said nervously. "Mel," I said with an incredible amount of restraint, "I will let you live." I meant it. Then I said, "If you feel that strongly about the idea that you risked your life over it, I'll use it."

The joke he was so passionate about was for a Professor sketch. The sketch had the Professor in a zoo. He is walking by the reptile house and he hears a tapping on the window. It's a snake tapping his teeth against the glass, trying to get his attention.

"What's the matter with you?" the Professor asks.

And the snake says, "You got to get me out of here. Please get me out of here."

The Professor says, "Why?"

"They're all snakes in here."

"What do you expect?" the Professor says. "You're a snake."

I did the joke on the show. Nothing — no laughs. Not a single one. Complete silence. "Mel," I said, "I will see you after the show." And I said it without the Professor's German accent with my two fingers pointed at him. From that point on, whenever someone in the Writers' Room suggested that we use an unpopular joke, we'd say, "You want to do the snake joke again?" Any bad joke became the snake joke.

Every Saturday night before the show, I

would take a one-hour nap in my dressing room with the door closed. No one was supposed to disturb me — it was strictly forbidden. Most of the time I would just close my eyes, take deep breaths, and try to relax. Mel would come by, open the door a crack, and whisper lines to me. Some of the lines had been vetoed in the Writers' Room. He was trying to get to me subliminally. Sometimes he had some good ideas and sometimes he had bad ideas — and a few times he actually succeeded.

One of the stories that gets told more often than any other about my relationship with Mel Brooks (and one that gets increasingly exaggerated each time it's told) has to do with how Mel found himself hanging out of the window of a Chicago hotel.

In between seasons of *Your Show of Shows* I went on tour as a "single" act. During the summer of 1950 I was booked at the Chicago Theater. I was originally scheduled for nine performances a day over a two-week period. The first show was at 10:00 a.m. and we would run until 11:00 p.m. The show was so well received, they didn't want to let me go and I was held over for six weeks. Dave came along with me for the engagement and since Mel had never been to Chicago and wanted to come, I invited him along as well to help out with some material.

Chicago was a rough city at the time, and Mel was — and still is — a little guy from Brooklyn. Not wanting to tempt fate, he sat around in the dressing room all day, waiting for me to finish my performances so that we could go out together.

I've never been able to eat between shows because a lot of food slows me down. I could never think well and consequently perform well if I'd put away a lot. I'd been snacking lightly all day, just a couple of bites of a sandwich after each show. By evening, I was starving. We were staying a few blocks away at the Palmer House in a suite on the eighteenth floor. I called ahead and ordered a salad, a nice, thick chateaubriand, a bottle of sparkling burgundy, asparagus, mashed potatoes with onions mixed in, and a piece of lemon meringue pie for dessert. Just placing the order made me salivate.

At the end of a long day I went back to the hotel, changed out of my suit and into a robe. Room service brought the meal right on schedule. I was just about to sit down, with the first piece of steak almost in my mouth, when Mel turned to me and said, "I wanna go out. I sat around the whole day in the dressing room and I wanna go out."

"Mel," I said. "You didn't have to stay there all day; you could've gone out yourself."

"Well, I was there — and now I wanna go out."

"Mel, I'm just sitting down to eat. We'll go out later."

The man was relentless. "C'mon Sid — for Chrissake! I want to go out now!"

"Mel," I said. "Please."

He wouldn't listen. "No, let's go out and eat, I want to get out." It was like a sketch right out of our show.

Finally, I just couldn't take it anymore. I put the knife and fork down, went over and grabbed him by the collar and his tush, and put him out the open eighteenth-floor window. "How far out do you want to go?" I asked. "Is that far enough?"

"Oh, no, I don't want to go out," Mel replied from somewhere over Chicago. "I'm out far enough."

"Are you sure?" I asked.

"I'm sure," came the reply.

Not for the first time, Dave grabbed me and calmed me down, and I pulled Mel back into the hotel room.

As people have told the story again and

again over the years, the floor of the hotel gets higher and Mel gets held farther and farther out the window. I think what makes this story endearing and not terrifying is that Mel knew that I was strong enough to hold him and that I would never drop him. We were two close friends who genuinely loved each other, and we had a relationship that was based on trust, affection, and his relentless attempts to piss me off.

Mel's first performance on the air was as an offstage voice. We were doing a parody of *Sudden Fear*, a picture that starred Joan Crawford. In the opening scene, a woman stroking a pet cat gets up to answer the telephone and receives what turns out to be a death threat. She hangs up the phone and steps backward onto the cat, which gives out an especially ominous screech. After looking through sound effects without much success, Max decided to give the job to Mel, who came up with a great scream and was given this weighty offscreen responsibility. He was fine through the rehearsals, up until the final dress rehearsal. When the stage manager gave Mel his cue, nothing happened. So between dress rehearsal and airtime, Mel got increasingly nervous. When the sketch aired, Mel was cued and gave an offstage cat scream that was worthy of Shakespeare.

Mel Tolkin and I took Mel Brooks under our wing. We even introduced him to our psychoanalyst. It was the '50s and everyone was into analysis. We also exposed Mel to classic literature, including Dostoevsky, Tolstoy, and Gogol, so we're probably indirectly responsible for his film version of *The Twelve Chairs*.

One Mel moment I'll always remember came at the 1957 Emmy Awards ceremony. Carl, Nanette, Pat Carroll, and I won Emmys and the show won for best series of one hour or more, but *The Phil Silvers Show* beat out *Caesar's Hour* for best comedy writing. Mel leapt up onto his table and screamed, "Coleman Jaacoby and Arnie Rosen won an Emmy and Mel Brooks didn't! That bullshit writers can win the award and geniuses like us would be denied! Nietzsche was right! There is no God! There is no God!" It was pure Mel. He really did know how to punch up a scene.

Max continued to add to the roster for *Your Show of Shows* throughout the life of the program with musicians, actors, and writers. The writers were always the best available and brought their own talents to the table.

When Lucille Kallen became pregnant (we can use that word now) and went off to have her baby, Max hired Neil Simon (who was known at the time as "Doc") and his brother Danny, who were a superb writing team. They had already written for the *Colgate Comedy Hour*. In their earliest days with us, the Writers' Room was so small they had to sit in the stairwell and pass in ideas.

The Simons were originally hired for a six-week engagement when Groucho Marx was supposed to be a guest on the show, but for some reason he did not materialize. Danny Simon (who later became a very good director) shared an apartment with Roy Gerber (who later became my agent). Danny's neatness versus Roy's sloppiness would later become the basis for Neil Simon's classic play, movie, and TV series, *The Odd Couple*.

I had seen a picture called *The Stranger*, in which Orson Welles, who also directed, plays a Nazi trying to hide in small-town America with Edward G. Robinson as the man who captures him. At the end of the picture there's a key scene involving a clock tower with giant revolving mechanical figures. I thought, what if these figures went awry. That would be a great premise for a sketch.

Max, however, didn't see the sketch's viability. "Max," I said, "there's something there. There's this beautiful clock and things keep going wrong. What if the pieces didn't work in sync with each other?" I had the brothers Simon rough out the sketch, and they came up with some wonderful material, which ultimately became one of our strongest and most successful sketches.

Doc and Danny wrote the wordless sketch for Imogene, Carl, Howie, and myself. We played mechanical figures that appear each hour on a large clock in the German village of Bauerhof. As we emerge from the clock on the hour, I hit the anvil, Carl hits my hammer, Howie pumps the billows, and Imogene cools the hammer with water. By the third hour the springs go haywire and Imogene begins to throw water in my face. As the mechanical figure, my first instinct is to hit her with the hammer. I exercise tremendous restraint to the audience's delight.

"It was comforting for the townspeople to come and watch that great clock," the announcer, Ed Herlihy, said as we moved forward to strike the bells. The hilarity of the routine, however, derives from the physical comedy. It really showed how smoothly the four of us worked as a team, and how often we all helped each other. All of the unscripted comedic action of the characters destroying one another led to the scripted punch line: "Anybody want to buy a ten-ton clock?"

Tony Webster, who had done great work for the *Bob and Ray* radio show, was also brought in to join the Writers' Room. Tony was the only member of the group that wasn't Jewish, so he was affectionately referred to as our "token goy." Joe Stein was also a top-flight writer; while he was with us he was also working on a play that became *Fiddler on the Roof.* He was and still is a very intelligent and funny man who made many valuable contributions. Joe joined us during the last two seasons of *Your Show of Shows* and stayed at my request through the transition to *Caesar's Hour.*

To the extent that the writers weren't treated with the utmost respect on *Your Show of Shows,* they certainly were on *Caesar's Hour.* I believed that the show began and ended with the writing, so no expense was spared in creating the most creatively friendly environment for the team. The latest incarnation of the Writers' Room, now in the Milgram Building, had desks and chairs and space to pace, because I always believed that writers need to move around to be creative. When they showed me a small room that was going to be the Writers' Room, I said no, writers have to walk. Some write sitting, some write leaning, and some write walking; everyone has a different style. I had them knock out a wall and we created a larger space. We put a plastic curtain across the room you could pull for privacy. Incidentally, when Neil Simon came up with the number twenty-three for the title of his play *Laughter on the 23rd Floor*, he got it by adding together the numbers eleven and twelve, which were the two floors the show had in the Milgram Building.

Behind the camera Lucille Kallen and Mel Tolkin had ended their long writing partnership. Lucille went to work with Imogene on her show, while Mel stayed with me, as did Tony Webster and Joe Stein. Carl Reiner was still a writer without portfolio, sitting in and making valuable contributions but not getting credited as a writer.

Mel Brooks, always unpredictable, had gone off to work on a play. He wasn't ready to be creative without the vibrant energy, cigar smoke, and deadlines of the Writers'

Room fueling him, only he didn't know that yet. Later that year he went on to write for Imogene as part of an attempt to save her show, which ended during its first season. Once Immy had a good script she was one of the most creative and inventive performers in history. She found pieces of business in every sketch. But Immy wasn't the kind of artist who could ask for what she wanted. She couldn't direct the development of a script.

With *Caesar's Hour*, probably as a reaction to the battles I had with Max over cutting the comedy for the sake of fifty-six choruses, I decreed that no musical number would go over four minutes unless it was part of a comedy sketch. There was no longer tension between musical productions and comedic sketches. Now comedy was truly king, with some sketches that ran for as long as forty minutes, which was most of the show. We were finally able to really tell a story.

With so many people gone, we needed to add to the writing staff, and in the first season of *Caesar's Hour* we added Aaron Ruben, Phil Sharp, Charles Andrews, and Shelly Keller. The truth was, every comedy writer in television wanted to be part of the show. It meant working with the top people in the business and being part of a team that allowed writers to shine. These were individuals in their twenties and early thirties who were the best and the brightest. Together we were creating new forms and styles of comedy. There was creative pressure and competition to make America laugh. In our room you couldn't get away with anything that was less than very funny. And there was no such thing as being too hip for the room.

Aaron Ruben, a top writer, was only with us for the first year of *Caesar's Hour*. He had written for Milton Berle and was very funny. Aaron was very industrious and approached his craft with a disciplined, businesslike attitude. He wanted ideas written down right away. He was a very well put together guy and went on to create both *The Andy Griffith Show* and *Gomer Pyle*, and also worked on *Sanford and Son*. That's some pedigree.

During the second season, although we lost Aaron, Joe Stein, and Tony Webster, we picked up even more writing firepower. That incarnation of the Writers' Room became the one most people remember.

Mel Brooks returned to the fold, as creative and as off-the-wall as ever. Mel had lost his way. He needed the guys around to give him competition and a kick in the ass. I gave him that. Figuratively and literally.

And we acquired a kid I'd heard about who was writing for Bob Hope, Larry Gelbart. Larry's father was a barber in Los Angeles, and as a teenager Larry would pitch jokes to people like Danny Thomas. Danny eventually hired him and he began a career as a comedy writer, spending five years with Bob Hope. What also drew me to Larry was that he'd played the saxophone in school. Like all of the other writers, he was also musical.

Larry was a studied genius. He never felt pushed. If he didn't get the right line or the right answer right away, he knew he would get it soon enough. Carl and Mel Brooks christened him the "Gentile Jew" because he wrote from "left to right" — his style was more deliberate and dialogue driven. The writer of *Tootsie* and *Oh God*, and the developer of the television version of *M*A*S*H*, among many great creations, Larry was a great idea man and had a brilliant ear for dialogue. "We were gifted, neurotic young Jews," Larry once said about the experience, "punching our brains out."

When new writers came in to work with me, I didn't put them under any pressure. I gave them two to three weeks to find their place and assimilate and get used to my style. With Larry, for the first two weeks he was there, I didn't speak to him, which apparently caused him some concern. He had no sense of how he was doing.

After the second show, as we were leaving Danny's Hideaway and waiting for cabs, I told him he was too young to be drunk and I kissed him on the lips. I validated him, and he was no longer worried about how he was doing as a writer, although kissing him on the lips probably gave him other things to worry about.

Neil Simon returned on a permanent basis and I wasn't about to let him get away this time. He was reserved and soft-spoken, and in the melee of the Writers' Room would communicate his ideas by whispering in Carl Reiner's ear. As quiet as he was, though, Neil was very proud of his work, and if challenged, would get very tough and protective. He was also developing *Come Blow Your Horn*, his first Broadway hit, while he was working for me.

Selma Diamond had been writing comedy since the radio days. She was a very intelligent, chain-smoking, street-smart woman, who was extremely funny, someone who gave as good as she got. She continued to provide the requisite woman's point of view in the Writers' Room. Selma later played the gravel-voiced wardrobe woman in *My Favorite Year*, and then was the first bailiff on the *Night Court* television series in the mid–1980s. She was also the never seen voice of Spencer Tracy's wife in *It's a Mad, Mad, Mad, Mad World*.

Selma had previously written for Goodman Ace, one of radio's biggest stars, a wonderful and very erudite man who was one of my idols. Goody wrote for one of my specials later on, and when we rehearsed the sketches he would turn around and face the wall, trying to simulate the effect of radio, as he listened to the dialogue. "What's all the laughter in between?" he would ask. "That's what *I* do," I told him.

Mike Stewart, who later went on to write *Hello, Dolly, Bye, Bye Birdie,* and *42nd Street*, became the Writers' Room scribe. Mike was an excellent writer who would also sit at the typewriter as the writers would pitch, miraculously capturing on paper all the ideas that I approved and turn them into a working script. I would nod as if it were a cattle auction acknowledging and accepting bids. I would say "put that down, that's good" to things that I liked. And amid the frenetic exchange of ideas and lines with guys pacing, standing on couches, and staring thoughtfully out the windows, Mike would type. A lot of stuff was coming at him; it would get to the point where somebody would say something and Mike would look at me and I'd shake my head. And another line would fly across the room, and Mike would look at me and I'd say, "Put it down." When I would turn to Mike and say, "Read it back," the other writers were often astounded that the yelling and screaming generated actual product. "You mean," they'd say, "there was something to read back?"

Once, after working late one night to finish a sketch, we broke for the evening. We left the script on the desk because we were going to polish it up the next morning. The cleaning woman came in, saw papers on the desk and put them in the trash, thinking it was scrap paper.

Mike was always the first one in every morning. He had already been looking for the script when the other writers got in the following morning. When he didn't see the script on the bare desk, he turned white. "Where's the script that was on the table?" he asked. No one knew. Mike looked for the cleaning lady, who told him the script was gone. It was a moment that would have crushed another man and another show. But without missing a beat, Mike sat down and retyped the entire sketch, word for word, dialogue, movement, stage directions, with nothing to go by except his memory. When I came in he told me what happened and showed me the newly typed sketch. He had not missed a word.

Like any good sports team, I was building a bench, a group of apprentice writers. I knew that not all the writers would stay with me, that some would be moving on to other projects, and I wanted to be ready. Gary Belkin and Sheldon Keller were part of that auxiliary group.

My brother Dave was also part of the *Caesar's Hour* Writers' Room. Though he was a member of the cast and did extra work in sketches, Dave would sit in on the Writers' Room and contribute lines and ideas. His sense of humor was sharper than mine. Dave was often the voice of the everyman when an arbiter was needed on how funny a joke or a sketch was. If he nodded when we talked out a skit, the voice of the people spoke in favor of it; if Dave shook his head, it was thumbs down. "If you interrupt us once more," Aaron Ruben once joked with him, "I'm going to have you demoted to cousin."

Dave was a very stabilizing influence whose mantra was "funny is money." He was always even-tempered and good-natured. He also kept the Writers' Room stocked with candy and would bring food in to feed an always hungry group of writers, which he would pay for out of his own pocket. After all those years, he was back in the restaurant business. Dave had brought in so many sandwiches that one day he handed a writer a piece of Swiss cheese and said, "my card."

Though Dave was often an extra in sketches, sometimes he wouldn't want to be. So when a writer would say, "that part would be perfect for Dave," my brother would turn to him and genially say, "Don't Dave me."

The six or eight writers sat around in a horseshoe and would pitch ideas, jokes, and dialogue. I sat in front of them as they pitched. Neil Simon once compared it to Jewish Indians on a bluff surrounding a wagon train. Larry Gelbart bought me a golden upholstered chair to serve as a throne for the Writers' Room, so I could preside in style.

The energy and pace were still frenetic. Chunks of plaster were knocked off the walls. Curtains were ripped to shreds. Images of Mel Brooks were hung in effigy by the other writers with some frequency. Mel's tapping on the shoes of a napping Larry Gelbart resulted in his own shoes being tossed out the window.

These guys had tremendous energy and creativity and would fight for lines. They got so worked up, they'd give each other hot-foots. Once they even set fire to my desk. They poured oil or some other flammable liquid on it and just set it on fire. I didn't even get angry. "Stop it, we have work to do," was all I said.

I was not without my own idiosyncrasies, like being fanatical about my suit staying pressed. On a hot day in the Writers' Room I would take my pants off and hang them up so that they wouldn't wrinkle. I was creating in my suit jacket, shirt, tie, and underwear. If I left the room during a lull, Aaron Ruben would push a Venetian-blind slat crooked. He knew I would come back and notice it immediately. It would get me so irritated, creativity would begin to flow with the adrenaline.

It wasn't always fun and games. Once the writers and I were sitting around for over an hour without coming up with any-thing. I was getting very restless; I always felt the pressure of the deadline. So I called Aaron Levine in the prop department and said, "Aaron, send me up an eight-foot Zulu spear. That's right. An eight-foot Zulu spear. Right away!" It miraculously arrived a half hour later. We all sat around the coffee table looking at it. Still no ideas. I then jumped up and threw this eight-foot Zulu spear across the room with all my strength. It stuck in the wall of the room and vibrated. "Now let's get to work," I yelled. I had to do something. And it worked! We came up with an Englishman sketch. Nanette and I parodied British royalty visiting a colonial tribe and interacting with the natives. We were dressed in white with pith helmets. A little native girl comes by and offers us flowers. I shoot the flowers. As the cavalry rides by in a cloud of dust, the prop men throw buckets of mashed potatoes at us. We stand stoically covered in dirt and mud. We had done our duty for the day.

When it came right down to it, we operated under a variation of the Three Musketeers ethic: all against each other, but all for the show. When push came to shove, what was best for the show was the main thing. As much as they all fought with each other, they respected each other.

I was still the one who drove the process.

If I didn't think something was funny or would work, I would press them to get something else going. I was still the fastest "no" in show business. If I didn't like something, I vetoed it quickly and dispassionately. We didn't have time to fool around. To avoid protracted arguments with the writers over whether an idea was good, now I had a metaphoric anti-aircraft machine gun with which I shot down ideas I didn't like. And those bullets couldn't have been more devastating — or more inspiring — to the writers whose ideas were mowed down if they'd been real.

I was always probing and dissecting the comedy to see if we could make something a little funnier, a little deeper, or a little more unexpected. What started out as a rubber tire sketch might turn into a soda fountain sketch. Because something in the process takes a sketch to a different, hopefully better place.

I was also learning the script as we wrote it, so I never had to take a script home to study. While I didn't memorize the dialogue word for word, I got the idea of what I wanted to say. But I knew every cue, the exact words, and what I needed to do with any other character. Carl was already in the Writers' Room regularly and Immy and Howie, and then Nanette, were also invited to the Writers' Room to listen to the sketches being developed so that they would be able to learn as well. During *Your Show of Shows*, we also had guest stars come in on Monday to discuss the proposed sketches to make sure they felt comfortable with what we were writing.

The work was throwing ideas around, literally. "I got it, Sid, how about this?" Sketches were built an inch at a time. Sometimes an idea fizzled out because it was not any more than a one-joke thing. Other times we would try and develop it. But if it took more than half an hour, there was usually something wrong. Maybe it was a one-joke thing, maybe we just hadn't got it right yet. Either way it didn't pay to take a chance on it. Other times, things started flowing quickly. An idea came and then another idea on top of that, and then a variation of that. The more variations you were able to get on a single idea, the better it was. It gave you much more room to move and there was a nice pace and a rhythm.

At the same time, a good idea was too precious to throw away, even if it didn't seem to be working. You couldn't let it go. Sometimes we came up with an idea that didn't fit me. We tried it on Carl, Nanette, or Howie. Many times I played it straight to Carl or Howie. It gave each of them the opportunity to showcase themselves as the top performers they were. I enjoyed letting them shine. I tried to spread the laughs. If you were the only one who's going to get the laughs in an hour and a half or even an hour, the show would get very boring very quickly. You can't be the whole macher. People resent it. My name was at the top of the show. If the show was funny, I was funny.

Speaking of funny, Milt Kamen was an excellent comedian in his own right. Carl discovered him, and he became part of the cast of *Caesar's Hour.* In addition to his other responsibilities, Milt would stand in for me during the dress rehearsals, and every once in a while he'd throw in a line that would remain in the show.

Milt made another creative contribution to the show and to show business in general. One day he brought in a young comedian he had seen working up in the Catskills, a short, redheaded kid from Brooklyn with big glasses, barely out of high school. "I'd like to introduce you to the young Larry Gelbart," he said. To which Larry quickly replied, "I thought I was the young Larry

Gelbart!" It was Woody Allen.

Woody wrote specials with Larry and myself. Woody was, not surprisingly, shy and quiet as a young man, but extremely smart and quick. The good ideas just kept on coming.

Once Woody got more confidence, when he wanted to say something, he made you listen, but never in a forceful way. It would always be "Sid, I'd like you to listen to this. I want you to hear this." It was wonderful. I said, "That's beautiful, Woody. That's great. Let's put it in."

One day I was sick with a stomach flu. I had to work but I didn't feel well enough to go to the office. So I sent a chauffeur to drive Larry and Woody out to my house in Great Neck. When they arrived, I felt like a steam, so I suggested that we work in the steam room I had in the house. So Larry and I got undressed and put on towels. Woody wouldn't get undressed. He said he couldn't be funny naked. So he wrote through the little glass window in the steam room. We would get an idea, then we'd open the door a little bit to hear what Woody had to say.

What we did is now considered classic comedy. Like classical music, it stuck to rules. (Today most people think classical music is Broadway show tunes.) The writers were all geniuses in their own way, and they each wrote differently. They had different styles, different ways of doing comedy. The writers also had the security to come up with terrible ideas and make their own mistakes. We all learned from each other. I was fortunate enough to be able to watch the brilliance develop and mature.

Our material worked, and still works today because we told stories about people. We had beginnings, middles, and ends. We created formats, concepts that transcended vaudeville and helped establish television as the preeminent source of entertainment in the world. The body of work we created has withstood the test of time. It has influenced and still continues to influence performers and artists today, because it was written by some of the greatest writers to ever put pencil to paper, and because we wrote about the human condition.

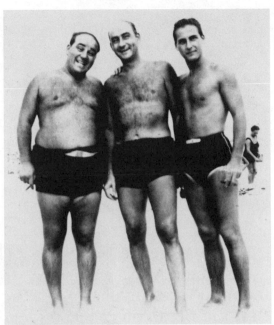

The brothers Caesar, Dave, Abe, and Sid, at the beach in our younger days.

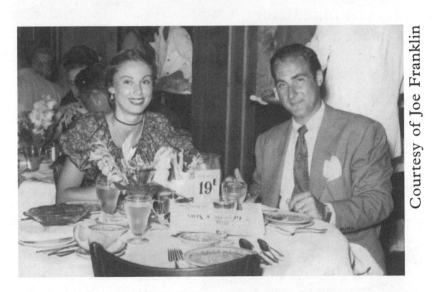

Florence and I enjoying dinner at the legendary Grossinger's Hotel in the Catskills in 1949.

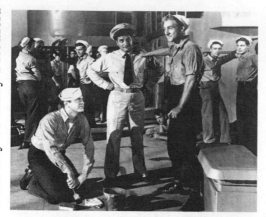

Tars and Spars, the movie version of our Coast Guard show, brought me to Hollywood.

The 1948 revue "Make Mine Manhattan" was my first big break on Broadway. This collaboration with Max Liebman immediately preceded our foray into television.

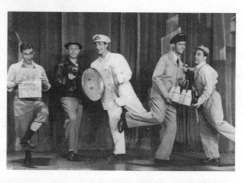

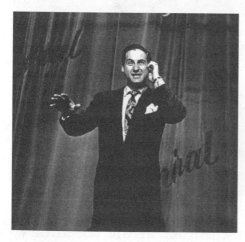

"The Five Dollar Date" was one of my earliest signature pieces. It brought together all of my talents, including double-talk. Here I am performing it on our first television program, *The Admiral Broadway Revue.*

278

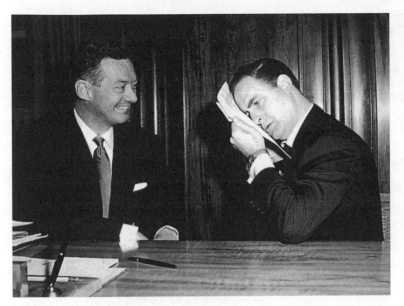

Here I am with the brilliant Pat Weaver, the future president of NBC, eyeballing my contract.

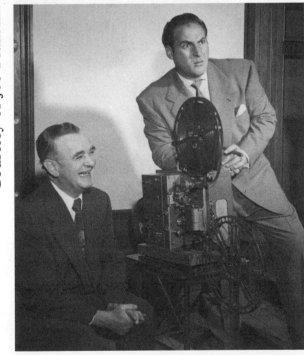

Max Liebman and I compare notes over a piece.

The very first Writers' Room, where
the magic began, with Mel Tolkin,
Lucille Kallen, and Mel Brooks.

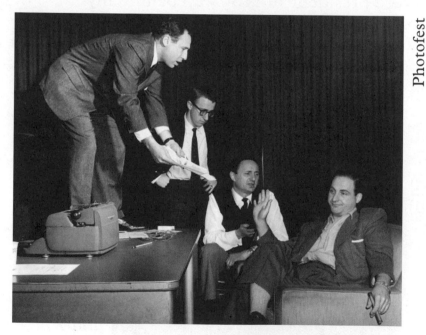

A later incarnation of the Writers' Room with a
typically animated Mel trying to sell an idea.
Woody Allen and Mel Tolkin look on.

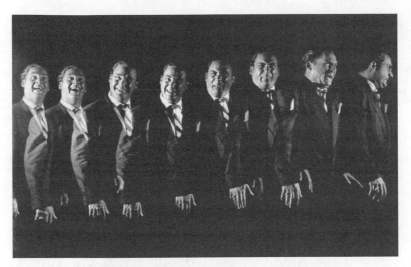

Famed photographer Phillipe Halsman took this time-lapse photograph of me changing moods.

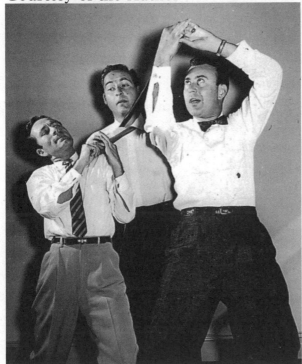

During our *Caesar's Hour* years, Howie Morris, Carl Reiner, and I were an unbeatable team. We took our comedy very seriously.

I was blessed to have two fantastic female co-stars. Imogene Coca and I connected on a visceral level and quickly became television's royal couple.

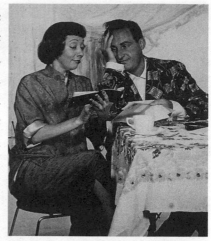

Courtesy of the Author

Courtesy of the Author

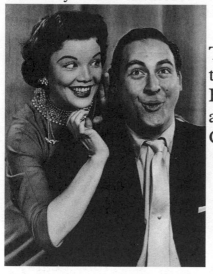

The beautiful and talented Nanette Fabray and me as Ann and Bob Victor, the Commuters.

Courtesy of the Author

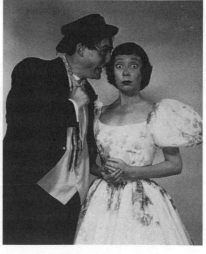

The Professor, the lovable but invariably wrong "expert" on every subject under the sun, with Imogene.

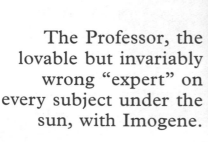

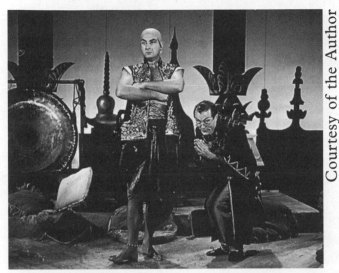

"How many times I gotta tell ya! No smokin' in the palace!" Our satire of *The King and I*.

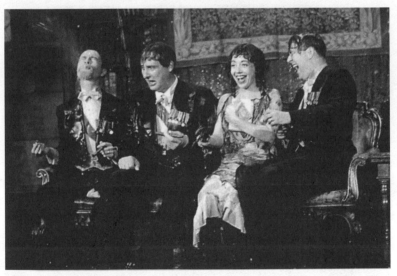
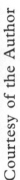

Howie, Imogene, Carl, and I as the unflappable Four Englishmen. This was a recurring sketch with the simplest of premises: We would sit on a bench and be confronted by any number of comic distractions. Nothing would move us. Here, with the cameras off, we were not so unflappable.

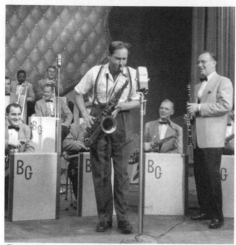

Playing with Benny Goodman, one of my idols, on *Caesar's Hour*, was one of the highlights of my musical and professional career. Comedy and music have so much in common and I often sought to combine the two.

Courtesy of Joe Franklin

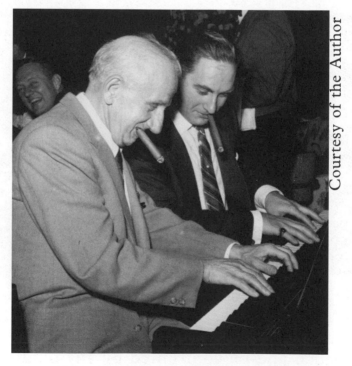

Jimmy Durante and I improvising together at a reunion of former NBC stars.

Chapter 8

THE HICKENLOOPERS and THE COMMUTERS

The best way to make contact with an audience is by doing something they do every day. A husband asking his wife, "Tell me what I said that was so wrong?" is not only universally understood and painfully funny, it is as germane to the husband/wife relationship today as it was fifty years ago, and as it will probably be a thousand years from now. A lot of men don't understand women. And a lot of women don't understand men. That's where the fun begins.

One of the very first sketches we began working on when we were getting ready to do *Your Show of Shows* was the domestic sketch. Domestic situation comedy had been a staple on radio for years. The Bickersons, Burns and Allen, and Fibber McGee and Molly were fixtures on the airwaves. But our weekly family feud between Charlie and Doris Hickenlooper was the first domestic situation comedy on television, predating Ralph and Alice Kramden and Lucy and Ricky Ricardo by more than two years.

Mel Tolkin and Lucille Kallen liked the notion of a recurring sketch about an ever arguing husband and wife, and we all liked the idea of starting the show with it every week. Charlie and Doris Hickenlooper, played by me and Imogene, were a mismatched couple who reflected the anxieties and frustrations of newlyweds. Charlie was the everyman, looking to get by, make a living, and live a quiet, enjoyable life. We left Charlie's status deliberately vague; he wore a suit and worked in an office. He wasn't rich but could afford a car. Sometimes he talked about an inventory; that, we felt, was specific enough so that people could identify. Doris was high-strung, ambitious, aggressive, slightly neurotic, and always trying to improve or change the very put-upon Charlie.

Doris: You know what the trouble is with you? You have no spirit of adventure! Don't you ever try something new, strange, unusual, a little bit off the beaten path, something a little weird, something you thought you'd never have anything to do with?
Charlie: (Looking at her straight in the eye

286

with a mean, measuring glance) Once.

Truth never changes. You still have to eat. You still fight with your wife. So starting each show with a domestic sketch was like shaking the audience's hands, making them feel at home. There is a certain timelessness to the arguments over money, friends, and the attention each spouse pays the other, which is still the basis for situation comedy and drama. Opening the show with a smaller sketch also allowed us to top it with something else later on. It provided us with a platform from which we could spring into the more outlandish sketches and keep the audience with us. First we would find the humanity and then we would find the wild comedy.

The beauty of the Hickenloopers sketches was that we were able to combine comedy with pathos. We were able to take real situations and then bend and twist that reality an inch or two so that the audience would see their own lives made fun of. We had the best of both worlds: we were able to use the situation comedy form and then mock it and take it to new levels.

I laughed at myself a lot and called myself a dummy. I set myself up as the clown, the fall guy, and the butt of the jokes. I was the self-assured guy who underneath it all was very insecure and keeps screwing up. I was everyone's brother, cousin, and uncle. In every downtrodden situation and every fight with my wife, even the smallest triumph got laughs and sympathy from the audience. Playing the goat and the victim was not easy for me because I was so big and strong looking. Practically every other comedian who practiced the technique of being the butt of the jokes was physically little himself, like Charlie Chaplin. It took a lot of acting on my part to pull it off and convince the audience to accept me in that role.

I came up with the name Hickenlooper after Senator Bourke B. Hickenlooper, who was one of the leading figures in the development of atomic energy. The choice had nothing to do with atomic energy. I just liked the name.

In those days most men got married right after the war, when they were twenty-three or twenty-four. They had gone through the war. They were no longer showering with five hundred guys or getting on a chow line. If the beans slipped into the Jell-O it was all right. They appreciated their own apartments and their wives. Unlike servicemen, they were in charge when they got married, or at least they thought they were.

288

We told couples they weren't alone in their feelings and showed just how ridiculous they could be. The audience understood the comedy and believed it, because people were either going through similar situations themselves or they were at least thinking about it. Believability was critical. If they didn't believe us, they wouldn't care. If I see something in a movie and I say to myself, "I don't believe it," I lose the whole plot. In these sketches, the audience could relate to the situation and take an interest in what went on. We also didn't preach. It was more important to get the laugh than to send the message. If there was a message there, we felt, it would follow naturally.

A couple could even disagree about what was funny. We once built an entire sketch around a couple fighting over whether a joke was worth laughing at, and the way Carl introduced that sketch was typical of our whole approach:

"Our opening sketch tonight deals with one of the problems of married life, of which, as we all know, there are many. Strangely enough, it's not always the big critical moments that cause tension between a husband and wife. Somehow, when a really important problem comes up, most of us can rise to the occasion and discuss it calmly and intelligently. But the little things are more difficult. It's the little things that cause all the quarrels. Little things like hanging stockings on the towel rack, or dropping cigar ashes on the rug. These are the insignificant molehills that become mountainous barriers between man and wife. Sid Caesar and Imogene Coca are no exception to the rule, when they have a difference of opinion."

Scene: Bedroom. Coca at dressing table brushing her hair. Sid is offstage.

Doris: 91, 92, 93, 94, 95 (She sighs with exhaustion, rests her arms) every night the same routine . . .

Charlie: (From offstage) What'd you say?

Doris: Nothing, nothing, you wouldn't understand. (Resumes brushing) Where was I? 96, 97, 98, 99, . . . 100! Well, that's that!

Charlie: (Coming in brushing his hair with military brushes) 213, 214, 215! (Puts down brushes) There! That's that!

Doris: Two hundred and fifteen!

Charlie: I didn't want to do a thousand because I've got a lot of work to do tomorrow. Goodnight, Dear. (They start getting into bed. Sid starts to laugh)

Doris: What are you laughing at?

Charlie: You know Harry Bells?

Doris: Of course I do.

Charlie: He was in the office today and told a joke that will knock you right off your chair. I got to tell you. It's the funniest joke I ever heard in my life. Listen to this. A cop is walking his beat . . . it's eleven o'clock at night. Suddenly he sees a young kid about eight years old, walking around the corner. A few minutes later, he sees the same kid walking around the corner again. For the next half hour, this kid keeps walking around the block, around and around. Never stops. So, finally, the cop goes up to him and says . . . "Look, Sonny, it's eleven thirty at night, you oughta be home in bed. Why do you keep walking around the block?" So the kid says . . . "I'm running away from home!" So the cop says, "Well, if you're running away from home, why do you keep going around the same block all the time?" and the kid says, "My mother told me never to cross the street!"

Doris: (A pause) Do we know the boy?

A huge argument ensues. The Hickenloopers argued about almost everything. Every argument seemed to escalate from the smallest thing. Charlie wanting a midnight snack, Doris worrying about her weight.

Charlie: Here we go. (Starts cutting the

roast) Boy, this looks delicious! I'll just take this end piece here . . . I know you don't like it . . . (Puts it on his plate) And here's a piece for you! (Starts to put it on her plate)

Doris: (Holding out a hand to stop him) No! Take it away!

Charlie: Why? What's wrong with it?

Doris: Nothing! I'm just not having any, that's all. Don't you understand English? I don't want any! Take it away! Eat it yourself!

Charlie: (Puts down knife and fork, and slams table) Doris, once and for all, there's something eating you up inside. I want to know . . . What's wrong with you?

Doris: (Bursts into tears) I'm on a diet! I'm starving. I haven't eaten a thing all day. All I had was half a glass of grapefruit juice and a raw carrot. I'm so miserable I could die! I'm hungry!

Charlie: *You're* on a *diet?* What for?

Doris: It'll make me healthier.

Charlie: You're healthy enough.

Doris: And it'll give me more energy . . .

Charlie: You've got enough energy.

Doris: And it'll make me slim and svelte and beautiful.

Charlie: How long will it take?

Doris: (Jumping up) You see? *That's* why I'm going on a diet! Because you make remarks like that!

Charlie: Like what? I didn't say anything. Look, I like you the way you are. As far as I'm concerned, you don't have to go on a diet. Forget the diet!

Doris: No! I made up my mind and I'm going to stick to it. It's just a matter of will-power and determination.

Charlie: All right, have it your own way. We'd better eat before everything gets cold. What are you going to eat?

Doris: I have my meal here.

Charlie: Where? There's nothing on your plate.

Doris: Yes, there is. Half an ounce of shredded carrot, a spoonful of yogurt, and one string bean.

Charlie: A whole string bean? Well, it's your life. If you wanna starve yourself, go ahead. Pass me the potatoes please. (She does. He helps himself) Pass me the gravy please. (She passes. He takes) The hot rolls, please. (Takes a slice) Butter please. (Smears a load of butter on a big chunk of bread, and starts to eat happily. Doris cuts up string bean into four tiny parts and eats it. Then she just sits and watches Charlie. He looks up) Why don't you eat?

Doris: I'm finished.

Charlie: You left something over.

Doris: That's the design on the plate.

Charlie: Oh. (He continues devouring food. Doris eyes him with hatred. He feels her watching him and tries to cover up his eating by turning away, bending down, sitting under the table with plate. When he comes up for second portion, he finds her eating) I thought you were finished. What are you eating?

Doris: The design on the plate! I'm starving!

Charlie: (Finally, in disgust) Look, this is ridiculous! I can't eat with you sitting there looking at me! Eat something. Take something to eat!

Doris: No!

Charlie: Look . . . how much weight do you wanna lose?

Doris: Thirty-five pounds.

Charlie: Thirty-five pounds! There won't be anything left of you. You're such a little thing.

Doris: I don't care.

Charlie: How much time are you giving yourself to lose thirty-five pounds?

Doris: Two days.

Charlie: Two days you're going to lose thirty-five pounds. You're a nut! You're really a nut!

Doris: Well, at least I won't be a fat nut!

Charlie: Why all of a sudden? Why do you

want to lose weight suddenly out of a blue sky?

Doris: I tried on my bathing suit this morning.

Charlie: So?

Doris: I can't get into it! (Gets up, goes to drawer, opens it, takes out a tiny garment) I want to be able to get into this.

Charlie: (Laughs) How much do you think you lost in one day?

Doris: We'll soon find out. (Takes out scale) I'm keeping the scale right here so I can weigh myself after every meal. (Steps on it, screams) Oh! I gained twenty pounds!

Charlie: That's impossible! You must be reading it wrong.

Doris: No I'm not. There must be something wrong with the scale.

Charlie: There's nothing wrong with the scale! Look . . . I'll show you. (He gets on the scale . . . There is a whirring sound ending with a boing)

Doris: You won a cigar. Sit down, I'll bring in dessert. (She goes)

Charlie: (To himself) I broke the scale! Boy! I must really have put on some weight! How do you like that! I didn't realize . . . hmmmm! Where's a mirror . . . (Stands in front of camera, looks himself over) Getting a little big. (Pats chin) My teeth are getting fat. I better do something. I'm going on a diet from now on.

Doris: (Entering with cake) Here's your favorite cake. Marshmallow chocolate fudge with banana filling and whipped cream butterscotch icing . . . I hope you enjoy it. (Pause) What's the matter?

Charlie: Nothing! Nothing's wrong!

Doris: I took the trouble to bake your favorite cake. You might keep a civil tongue in your head!

Charlie: My tongue is too fat to keep in my head. I'm getting fat all over. I'm going on a diet.

Doris: (Laughs) You're going on a diet!

Charlie: What's so funny about that? I'm not going to eat any of that stuff. (Sticks finger into cake . . . licks fingers)

Doris: You're not going to eat any more desserts like this? That'll be the day! (Does same business)

Charlie: I wouldn't touch this cake for a thousand dollars. (Same business)

Doris: You'd eat it for a penny. (They both dive into the cake and continue arguing)

Restaurants were always popular venues for sketch comedy. Once we played a couple trying to decide how to tip at a fancy joint. When the check arrives, we start to deliberate based on the white tablecloth, the maître d', the number of waiters and busboys. I am doing all the calculations on the tablecloth, writing all over it. I finally come up with the right number for the tip: eight cents.

Carl did a wonderful job as the intimidating headwaiter who can't be satisfied. I start peeling bills off my bank roll. Nothing. No matter how many bills I give him, he still stares at me condescendingly. No thank you, nothing. I write out a few personal checks. I toss him my wristwatch and cuff links. Immy gives him her earrings. I even offer him my insurance policy. Still no reaction. Immy and I finally flee, with Carl yelling after us, "Cheapskate!"

In another sketch, Immy played a frantic wife who believed she was the object of desire of every man who saw her.

We are barely out of a cab to go into a restaurant and already she is starting in. "Did you see him," she whispers. "He was looking at me. Did you notice? The entire trip, the cab driver was looking at me."

"He's gone now," I reply calmly.

We go into the restaurant, and she starts in again, and you know she believes it: "Did you see how the headwaiter is looking at me!"

"Really?"

We sit down at our table. "That man is looking at me."

I look back and the headwaiter, played by Carl, is reading the newspaper. "Are you going to stand for that?" she demands.

I reluctantly walk over to Carl. "Excuse me, my wife thinks that you're looking at her."

"I'm reading the paper," he calmly replies.

I apologize and invite him to dinner.

Imogene was not the most beautiful woman in the world, but she acted like she was. She was able to pull that off magnificently, playing the character as if she was as desirable as Greta Garbo.

One of the writers came in one Monday morning and said, "Did I have an experience at a party this weekend, a guy and his wife started fighting because she had smashed the car into a funeral home, and he just found out she forgot to pay the auto insurance premium." By the end of the day, we had a complete sketch for Imogene and me, based on that idea, called "Breaking the News." It's another one of my favorite sketches because it is so well balanced, and you can see Charlie slowly exploding.

Doris: Hello, Mother? Where have you been?

I've been trying to get you for *hours*. I just had to talk to somebody. Well, I had a little accident with the car. Nobody was hurt. But I don't know how I'm going to tell Charlie! You know how madly in love he is with that silly car! Well, I don't know how it happened — I was driving along Elm Street and I was passing by Flora's Millinery Shop and she had an Empress Eugenie hat in the window and I was thinking: "My goodness, are *those* things coming back?" And I guess it just took my mind off the driving for a *minute,* and the next thing I knew I went right through the window of Jim Grady's liquor store! Yes, the bottles and everything. Well, the car is in pretty bad shape. It's in the garage now — he's going to call me later and let me know what the damage is. Oh — I hear Charlie coming . . . I'll call you later, Mother. Good-bye. (Hangs up, straightens herself, and puts on a big smile) (Charlie comes in looking beat)

Doris: Hello, you darling boy! You look wonderful today! How do you feel?

Charlie: Miserable! What a day! Those people at the office — I'm telling you I can't *stand* it anymore! Such incompetence! Such carelessness! If there's one thing I can't stand, it's a careless person! A person who doesn't watch where he's going! I could kill a person like that. Can you imagine somebody just carelessly tripping over a wastebasket and putting a dent in it? Can you imagine? That's about a two-dollar damage! Just because of carelessness!

Doris: Why don't you relax, dear. I have a wonderful dinner for you. Everything you like.

Charlie: I can't eat now! I'm so nervous and upset — I couldn't eat a thing! I think I'll take the car and go for a drive.

Doris: No! No! Just sit down and have dinner.

Charlie: Believe me, I can't eat now. I'll go for a drive in the car. It'll relax me.

Doris: No! Please. The dinner will get cold. Why don't you relax here. After you have something to eat, you'll feel better.

Charlie: Well, maybe you're right. Maybe if I have something to eat, I'll settle down a little.

Doris: Of course you will. You'll feel much better after you eat.

Charlie: (Picks up fork and raises food to his mouth — then throws it down) It's no use — I can't eat! I'm going for a drive, clear my head.

Doris: No! No! No! (Pushes him back in chair) I don't think it's a good idea! Just try to forget about it. Look you know what I made for you, your favorite dish — kidney stew with lobster sauce.

Charlie: All right. (Starts to eat) I guess I'll feel better after dinner. Mmm, this tastes good.

Doris: (After a pause) Poor Jim Grady.

Charlie: Who?

Doris: The man who owns that liquor store on Elm Street.

Charlie: What happened?

Doris: Someone drove their car right through his window.

Charlie: Drove a car through the window? You're kidding! Was anybody hurt?

Doris: No, nobody was hurt. But it was pretty messy. Especially the car!

Charlie: Oh boy! What a store to smash up . . . A liquor store! What a smashup *that* must have been! I'll bet it was a woman driver! (Doris nods) Sure! That's what I thought! Some crazy idiot woman driver! But I don't blame her so much! She shouldn't be allowed to drive a car! She must have a crazy idiot *husband!* Any guy who lets his crazy wife drive a car is crazy!

Doris: Yes, I guess it is the husband's fault!

Charlie: Sure it's the husband's fault! Letting a wife like that drive the car! I'm telling you, you're not safe walking in the street anymore! Can you imagine what the damage is going to cost him? A liquor store?

301

Wow, that car must be soaked with alcohol! It's gonna cost him a pretty penny. A very pretty penny! About five million pretty pennies!

Doris: (After a pause) I've been thinking. I don't think I'll get that fur coat after all.

Charlie: What?

Doris: I don't really need it. I still have my raccoon.

Charlie: What are you talking about? We've been putting money aside every week for two years, and now we have enough to buy the coat, and you're gonna get it. Remember when I bought the car, you were ashamed to ride in it because you weren't dressed up enough? You said the car looked better than you did. Well now you'll have a new fur coat and you'll look just as good as the car. Of course, you won't have hubcaps. So you're going to get the coat.

(They eat again)

Doris: Well, maybe we won't have to take a vacation this year.

Charlie: What? What do you mean no vacation? You know how I look forward to that all year. What's the matter with you? You talk as though we're broke! Thank goodness I have a very good business. If only those stupid idiots in my office wouldn't be so careless! Oh! I see purple every time I think of it! It makes me choke! I can't forget about it! (Gets up) Come on . . . Let's go for a drive in the car.

Doris: Wait! Wait!

Charlie: Wait for what?

Doris: No! I don't think we should go for a drive tonight!

Charlie: Why not?

Doris: Well . . . I might as well tell you . . . I sent the car to the garage for repairs. (Continues talking as Charlie says . . .)

Charlie: What kind of repairs?

Doris: You know Joe's Garage . . . They're so handy . . . Huh? Oh. Well . . . Just a few minor repairs.

Charlie: But just last week I had a thousand mile checkup!

Doris: Well they couldn't have checked it very well.

Charlie: What's wrong? Is the carburetor out of order?

Doris: Probably.

Charlie: The brakes don't hold?

Doris: I wouldn't be surprised.

Charlie: Is a wheel out of line?

Doris: They're all out of line. The whole thing sort of . . . curves . . . The doors . . . The glass . . . The tires . . . The upholstery . . . Spots . . .

Charlie: (The light begins to dawn. He

screeches) You! You went through the store window! You're the crazy woman! And I'm the crazy husband! You! A whole liquor store! The bottles, the window!

Doris: And the fixtures!

Charlie: The fixtures!

Doris: Well Jim Grady was very nice about it. He wasn't nearly as mad as Doc Fletcher!

Charlie: Who is Doc Fletcher?

Doris: The man who owns the drugstore across the street.

Charlie: The drugstore too? You went through the drugstore?

Doris: (Indignant) Well, I had to back out of the liquor store!

Charlie: Sure! Of course! You had to back out! Oh and a liquor store and a drugstore smashed up!

Doris: (Whimpering) It was just an accident. It could have happened to anyone.

Charlie: (Controlling himself, gritting his teeth) All right, all right. There's nothing we can do about it now. Thank goodness I was smart enough last week to remind you about sending that check to the insurance company. It was just lucky that we renewed the insurance just in time. Lucky, lucky me! Because if I didn't remind you to send the check, boy, we'd be in hot water! But luckily, I reminded you. So you must have sent the check. Boy am I lucky. I'm a pretty lucky boy! Because if you didn't send the check . . . (Starts to groan, make noises, walks back and forth, mutters) I'm afraid to ask. I'm not gonna ask. I can't ask. (Clears his throat) Did you? You . . . Did . . . You sent . . . You . . . Did . . . Did you send . . . The check . . . to the Insurance Company?

Doris: (Grins and nods "yes")

Charlie is beyond relieved and hugs Doris.

The censors dictated that couples slept in separate beds, as was the norm for married couples on television for years to follow. If you sat on the bed, you had to keep one foot on the floor. In one sketch, I was the husband who couldn't fall asleep. I had a big meeting the next morning and was anxious. I spent the night tossing and turning, flopping my pillow, tossing my blankets, all the while watching my wife sleeping the sleep of angels.

I would make noises and try and get her to wake up. "Doris, I can't sleep."

"Why don't you take a couple of sleeping pills?"

"Where are they?"

"In the medicine chest."

I take the pills and begin dancing around the bedroom. I found a piece of business during rehearsal that was based on "Piccolo Pete," a popular song and I animatedly say: "Did you ever hear Pete go tweet tweet tweet on his piccolo? No?"

Immy wakes up again. "Did you take the sleeping pills?"

It turns out I took some pep pills. I then take the sleeping pills and begin falling asleep and waking up in rapid intervals. The sketch ends when Immy takes the pep pills and we start dancing around the bedroom together.

There comes a time in every marriage, however, when talking stops. And even in the best marriages, there are many different ways to argue. There's silent arguing, there's noisy arguing, there's grunting arguing, there's the two-second incomprehensible hollering. There is a definite loss of eye contact, and all you hear are grunts and growls and the loud banging of silverware. The best argument sketches had no dialogue at all. In one of them, I showed her how lousy her cooking was. I picked up the saltshaker and her eyes told me that she didn't want her food seasoned. I took off the top and poured out all the salt to show her just how bad I thought it was. Then I had to eat it. I cut off a piece and started to chew it. She began to giggle. People loved to laugh at themselves over these kinds of sketches.

We crafted another sketch where Immy and I got into such an intense argument that there was just noise. No talking, just slamming. Put the dish down — bang! Put the fork down — bang! I put a glass of water down and broke it. We were so mad, we couldn't say word one to each other. We showed the crazy side of married life. We were so mad at each other neither of us could speak to the other one.

The payoff was that after three days of silence, I finally spoke and asked her, "Do you remember what we were arguing about?" And the irony was that neither of us could. I said "I think we oughta talk because we're gonna run out of money if we keep breaking dishes." That's where the poignancy comes in as the husband thinks: "What am I doing? What was so important? I'm making myself miserable for nothing. I want to come home, I want to have some food, and I want to have some light conversation without it turning into the Crimean War."

Those everyday arguments were the core of every argument-related domestic sketch. What set us apart was that we weren't afraid of showing the emotional and crazy sides of married life.

★ ★ ★

When we moved to *Caesar's Hour*, the domestic sketches were still a mainstay, still the best way to draw the audience in. With Imogene gone, the Hickenloopers were replaced by "The Commuters," three couples who lived in the suburbs. While the Hickenloopers rarely went beyond me and Imogene, the Commuters were about three couples: Nanette and I played Ann and Bob Victor, Carl and Howie played my best friends George Hansen and Freddie Brewster, with their wives played by either Pat Carroll, Shirl Conway, Virginia Curtis, Sandra Deel, or Ellen Parker.

That wasn't the only difference. By this time the post–World War II economic boom had really taken effect. People had money, and all over the country they were moving out to the suburbs. We started to focus on the problems people had with upward mobility and keeping up with the Joneses.

An early sketch on *Caesar's Hour* called "The Small Apartment" showed the Victors before they left the city. Though Carl and Howie had already moved to the suburbs, Nanette and I still lived in a room-and-a-half apartment with a Murphy bed coming out of the wall and a kitchen that's just about as long as your arm. It was so small that Nanette could cook and set the table in the living room without taking a step.

The most ridiculous thing you could do in that small apartment — where no two chairs matched and you could barely get a tray out of the kitchen without spilling the food because the doorway was so narrow — was have a turkey dinner on the tiny telephone table, which is what we did. We kept working out bits the audience would believe, from Carl bragging about having a whole closet just for his belts to our closet exploding from all the furniture we had stuffed in it. Everyone in New York has had an experience like that.

Because the times had changed and because our budget could handle it, the Commuters sketches were grander than the Hickenloopers. Once they got to the suburbs, Bob and Ann were always going out or entertaining guests. We could afford more people onstage and more sets and props, so we used them. In one sketch we had a party, and Nanette kept inviting more and more people. We wanted to make the party look crowded, so we brought in a lot of extras. But with the camera pulling back, it never looked crowded enough. So we hired more extras.

Finally Leo Morgan said, "Enough! No more extras! You're hiring people like crazy!"

I realized what was happening and asked Clark Jones, "Why are you pulling the camera back? I want to fill the scene up." "Why didn't you tell me?" he replied. "I just thought you wanted more actors!" We put up another wall to create the effect of a packed party. The sketch also had a priceless moment of Howie taking a nap on the bed. As more guests came in, they kept throwing their coats on the bed. When we went looking for Howie, he was buried underneath a high pile of coats and yelling for help.

People were very proud of their new homes and the care they put into them. So after the Victors moved to the suburbs, we did a sketch about our brand new white carpet, "from a Himalayan nanny goat." We are showing the carpet off to our friends one evening during a rainstorm. They are allowed to look at it but are strictly forbidden to walk on it unless they take their shoes off first. When Howie makes a move to step on the carpet, I literally scoop him up and carry him under one arm across the rug. The steps we take to protect the carpet keep escalating. Carl finally shows up late. He enters through the kitchen door. Always the gentleman, he has the courtesy to remove his shoes before he walks on the carpet. But his rain-soaked black socks bled through onto the carpet, leaving near-heart-attack-producing footprints on the no longer pristine white carpet.

One night in the Victors' kitchen, the women are playing Scrabble, trading letters, while the boys are playing gin. Howie and I go to make a quick cup of coffee for the guests. Coffee turns to cocoa with cookies. Carl joins us and the three men start to make sandwiches. We begin playing with a piece of cheese and suddenly we're piling our sandwiches with ham, artichokes, peppers, oysterettes, toast, scrambled eggs, lobster, chow mein, shredded cabbage, cucumbers, and chutney.

Nanette is doing a slow burn as all of us have taken over the kitchen. It's now one in the morning, and the other couples leave. It's just Nanette and me and one big mess. I nonchalantly ask Nanette to take care of it and she explodes. I in turn tell her, "I happen to be the husband. I have never evoked my husbandry here. I am the commander in chief here. I am in command of every room here, including the garage.

You shall be the good wife and clean up, and I shall go to sleep, like a good chiefy." As I lay in bed, Nanette dumps all the dishes on top of me. "I was sure I won that argument!" is all I can say.

When we weren't eating at home, we were eating at nice restaurants. One restaurant sketch revolved around the inevitable awkwardness of how three couples share the check. Carl and Howie and their wives conveniently go to the rest rooms and the waiter hands me the check. I study it, look at him, and ask, "You sure this is our check — and not a check for the nation?"

I pay the check and tell Nanette, "When the boys come back, we'll divvy it up."

Bob: The check inevitably arose and I paid it.
George: Here's $10. That should cover it.
Bob: Well there's about $40 still sticking out.
George: This is a clip joint. They're not getting another penny from me. That's all they get from me!
Bob: They're not me. I am they! I bought out they!
(Carl starts to itemize the bill: "Us, they, and you all." I get queasy when I learn that escargot is snails.)

George: There's a $12 discrepancy.
Bob: Are you saying I discreeped with $10?

As it turns out, there is a $12 cover charge for the music. We are all friends again.

Another sketch about going out has Nanette and I getting all dressed up to go to a charity ball. Unfortunately that's the last she sees of me. When Nanette looks to dance, she finds me and the boys playing cards. She asks me to dance and I say, "What do you mean, dance? We're married. What's the percentage?" Nanette gets mad and winds up dancing wildly with another man. I cheer the dancing on until I realize that it's Nanette. When we get home she tells me that all she wanted to do was dance. I say, "Why didn't you just ask me?" An incredulous Nanette keeps saying the words "ask him" over and over and walks away shaking her head. I realize she is right. Without saying the words out loud, I mouth, "I'm sorry" and she falls into my arms. I put a record on the hi-fi, and we dance.

One of my favorite sketches was "The Fur Coat." Nanette and the other wives go shopping where she buys an expensive mink and then has to figure out how to break the news to me. When I come home, she kisses me passionately. I know something is wrong. I start to assess, based on the kiss, the level of disaster.

Bob: You smashed the car?
Ann: No.
Bob: It's just love?
Ann: Can't a married woman kiss her husband for no reason?
Bob: That wasn't a marriage kiss, that was a money kiss. That was a $300 kiss.

She has made roast beef with lemon meringue pie for dessert. Nanette lights my favorite cigar and then comes out of the kitchen wearing the new mink coat.

When I see the coat, I start to cry. The stagehand blew camphor in my face to induce the flow of tears. Nanette falls into a beautifully improvised monologue about how we will save money because this is the only gift she will ever want. She is giving me the time to cry and develop my part. While she is talking, all I do is cry. There is a tight shot of my face as I tear. "I got no money, lady" is all I can say, over and over.

Ann: Now, look, the coat cost $725. Now, the coat's going to last me at least ten years. So over a period of ten years, that's

314

just twenty cents a day.

Bob: All right, here's twenty cents. Catch me every morning for the next ten years, you get the coat.

Ann: If we don't go to Bermuda this year, we'll save $500.

Bob: If we don't go to Paris, we'll save $1,000!

Nanette leaves the house, and I don't know where she is. I am overcome with worry. When she comes home, I go and get the coat for her. "It'll mean giving up a few things, like cigars and water, but it's worth it."

Now she doesn't want it, but when the other couples come in and the wives are wearing fur coats, Nanette changes her mind. She'll take the coat. I give up. "Let's take a walk around the Joneses' house to show that we're keeping up."

We even did a sketch about whether couples should wear their wedding rings, when Bob didn't want to:

Bob: I don't believe in men wearing jewelry. What is a ring? It's circular, it's gold, it goes around and around forever, like love.

Ann: That's beautiful.

Bob: That's baloney, which is also round . . . It's different for a woman. When I walk down the street and see a woman, the first thing I look at is the finger on her left hand, so I know whether to say, "Good morning" or *"Hello there!"*

Speaking of rings, we did a domestic sketch based on the fact that many a man could not afford a nice engagement ring (or any ring at all, for that matter) for his fiancée when they first got engaged, and years later wanted to surprise his wife with something nice.

Building on that premise, I buy Nanette a nice ring as a gift for our anniversary to replace the little chip I got her when we were first married. I proudly tell Carl about the gift.

He says, "Can I see it?"

"Sure," I say, showing him the ring.

"What did you pay for it?" he asks.

"What's the difference, it's a three-karat ring; $3,500."

"$3,500 for this?"

"Yeah, why, what's wrong with that?"

"I saw the same ring in another store for $3,000. Same ring. Same karats, same kind of cut."

So at our anniversary party I give her the ring and the guests all applaud. Now I know when she does the dishes, she always takes her ring off and puts it on the sink. So she gets distracted and I take the ring, and I'm going to the other jeweler and I'm going to get the same ring for $3,000. She comes out of the kitchen hysterical. She can't find the ring — "Oh my God, I lost the ring! You just gave it to me and I lost it!" Now I am beside myself. Holy cow, what did I do! And I'm looking at Carl and Carl is looking at me.

"Be strong," Carl says.

"I'm not that strong," I tell him.

When I see what I am putting her through, turning the house upside down, I say forget the $500. I pretend to find the ring under a seat cushion. "Hey," I say, "I found it! It was under here." That turned out to be one of the best sketches we ever did. It's simple and reflected the connection between husbands and wives.

Life is full of conflict. There will always be the opportunity to fight. If it's something that's very important, you sit down and talk to your spouse: "Sweetheart, I'm sorry that I did this and I realize that it's part my fault and it's part your fault too. So we both have to work out which way we want to handle this."

It was this attention to the human connection that made the domestic sketches so successful.

Chapter 9

THE ART OF SKETCH COMEDY

A sketch is like a small play. You have to tell some of the story up front to ensure that the audience is with you and knows what is happening. In a sketch, in the first ten to fifteen seconds, you have to know who each character is, why he is there, what he does, and what his relationship is to everybody around him. That's so the audience can understand how you're playing the character. You have to establish characters because that's where your comedy comes from. If someone says something out of character, you don't believe him and consequently you don't believe the sketch.

Most importantly, you need to tell a story. That's what delivers the comedy. Comedy is exaggerated truth. I never believed you should have a joke hanging out there all by itself. Even if it gets a big laugh. The joke needs to have something to do with the sketch. If it doesn't connect, don't do it.

It's a distraction and it takes you away from what you want to say. Neil Simon has said that most of his comedies are dramas in disguise because there is something at stake for the characters.

Comedy reflects the culture that it comes from. There once was, "Good evening, ladies and gentlemen. Welcome to the show." It's now hi, how's everybody doing? That's a subtle but very significant change. There's a style, a level of refinement that is gone. The language used today would not in anyone's wildest dreams have been used on television when we were starting out. Who would have ever guessed that "motherfucker" would become accepted as just a regular word. In fact, it's too often used as a crutch instead of actual funny lines or insights. If you're going to use that kind of language in ordinary conversation, what do you say when you're mad? Nothing. Because you've said it all.

There's a certain point where each culture accepts art in a particular way and decides what the standard is. No one person decides anything. If society likes it, it's in. Then the culture will drop something, either because it has latched onto something else or because that item has simply become tired.

In the late '40s and early '50s, there were

319

strict rules about what kind of comedy you could do. You could do a generic politician, but no one specific. You couldn't touch religion at all, and you couldn't go anywhere near sex. You could get away with "Wow, she's some looker," but you could never say, "Would you look at the hooters on that broad!"

Working under almost Victorian censorship made us work a little harder, and it drove us to be more creative. You couldn't say "damn" or "pregnant." The hottest word we could say was "heck." No one on television at that time ever needed to go to the bathroom. We did a prison sketch without dirty language. Politics, sex, sponsors, specific corporations were off-limits, which made it even more of a challenge to be funny. We also stayed away from topical humor, which I always believed was for wrapping tomorrow's fish in.

We couldn't go for a cheap joke or a shock joke. We had to be funny on our own. These limitations made us think. Instead of going for the easy laugh with profanity or an off-color remark, we always had to be creative and come up with something that was both funny and clean. We drew from real life. Things aren't funny, people are funny. We would never have a guy walk into a room with a piece of toilet paper stuck to his heel. We had to be subtle.

I believed then, and still do, that if you're an entertainer, especially a comedian, you can be satirical, but you can't engage the government head-on. There is a very thin line between being a politician and an entertainer. You can't knock the entire system because you never really know what's going on inside and why certain decisions were made. My job is to make you laugh and make you happy. My personal opinion is my own. I don't want to know how you vote, and you don't need to know how I vote. And neither of us needs the Supreme Court in our bedroom.

In the movies in the '30s and '40s, you didn't need to see a naked woman to get you excited. Just seeing two people sitting on the same bed, even with all four feet on the floor, could get you going. You would see a man and a woman kiss and then the camera would meld into miles of meadows, ocean waves crashing, or trees waving in the wind. The rest was left to your imagination, and that's what made it evocative. The reason radio was exciting is because the audience had to think, they had to work to get that feeling of ecstasy. They had to work to paint the picture in the mind's eye.

Our comedy was of the same vintage.

The illusion was that little girls were made of sugar and spice and everything nice. At that time, if you went out with a girl, and you went to the movies, it took you an hour or an hour and a half to get your arm around her. By the time you finally got your hand around her shoulder, your whole arm was numb. You didn't know if you were feeling her breast or her shoulder. But you were holding her, and that was the big deal.

When we did a satire on the Lux Radio Theater, we called it "The Lust Video Theater." The censors wouldn't allow that. They thought it was too offensive. They made us call it "The Nice Video Theater." They wouldn't even let us use the bing-banging sound that the old Lux radio show began with. We would put in words we knew would get cut out so that we could trade them off for others that we wanted in. Movie directors do the same thing today in dealing with the MPAA ratings board.

Our battles with censors and sensitive sponsors went back to the early days. On the Admiral show, we wanted to do a sketch about a guy bringing home a television set. He was so excited, so proud that he could bring a TV set home, that he started telling his wife to rearrange the furniture in the apartment trying to find a place for it. I was pantomiming walking around the apartment lugging the big set, and then pantomimed pulling all the furniture out. The agency representative said, "You can't do that. You're making fun of television." They made us pull the sketch on Friday, so there wasn't enough time to write a replacement. I wound up improvising a sketch about a man waking up in the morning. He brushes his teeth, and as he rinses his mouth, he swallows the gargle water. When he starts to shave, he keeps trying to get his sideburns even, cutting from side to side and measuring them, until all of a sudden he's bald.

When I did a sketch of a boy looking at the pretty girls at his first dance, I found a piece of business during rehearsal that I really liked. The boy is so flabbergasted he's talking to a girl that his tongue keeps falling out of his mouth in awe. The censors wanted me to cut that part. They thought it was overtly sexy, but I stood my ground. "It's a kid at a dance," I told them. "You can fire me if you want, but it's not going out." Over forty years later, I did the same routine on *Late Night with Conan O'Brien*, and the tongue wagging got the biggest laugh from the audience; even though against a '90s backdrop it was a very tame piece.

Much of comedy today comes out of a mold. "Let's do a show exactly like that, only different." There are great shows out there, and there are ones not to my choosing. I am actually quite fond of *Everybody Loves Raymond*. It is comedy based on truth. They don't have to go that far to get the laugh. There used to be broadcasting. Now there's what everyone calls narrowcasting. There are entire stations devoted to news, movies, or comedy. There are a number of stations devoted to business and finance. There are country-western singers who are extremely popular in four or five states and practically unknown beyond. And now on the Internet you can go and look up whatever you want. But the more technical we get, the dumber we get. It's a different world. The values are altogether different. When you get to the point where a character can have sex with an apple pie, you've just lost it.

I have always believed that working dirty is a crutch. If you open that door, you begin to depend on it. Once your mind goes that way, so does your comedy. If you know you can't or won't do that, your mind goes in a different direction. As an artist, I have to say it is offensive to me. I couldn't say a dirty word in front of an audience if you paid me. It's different if you're with a bunch of guys at a roast or a smoker. Behind closed doors, anything goes. But if there are women and children in the audience, no thank you, no way.

People respect comedians who don't resort to the cursing crutch. But they are treated in a different way. Of course, there are times when profanity is used to advance the comedy. That's when it's true. If a bunch of marines are sitting down to eat, "Hey, you want to pass the gosh-darn butter?" doesn't do it. That's when profanity is supposed to be used because it adds to the character and the flavor of the scene.

It is often said, by people inside and outside the business, that Richard Pryor opened the door for comedians to curse. Which is not true. Richard Pryor didn't open the door. When he cursed it meant something. It was part of the act and it was appropriate in the context. The same was true of *All in the Family*. It was very controversial for 1972; it involved a lot of sensitive issues. But using real-life language worked because it was believable.

I have always adhered to the cardinal rule of believability. If I didn't believe in the sketch, I didn't believe in the characters, and I wasn't going to do it well. And if the audience doesn't believe you, they lose interest.

We developed composites that had characteristics of people, but never enough so that anybody would ever be offended. We knew what we were doing — taking little bits and pieces of people and melding them together. We never personalized it. You could never look at a sketch and see someone's wife in it. The job was not to offend, it was to entertain. Which is unlike comedy today, where too often the goal is to offend, and if you have entertained, it's an unexpected bonus.

Once you start to like the character, you believe in him and he entertains you, and that's it. You're a hit. Comedy is as much about storytelling as it is anything else. It is drama and character driven. Jackie Gleason understood this with *The Honeymooners*. The chemistry between the characters drove that show. You believed that everything Art Carney did as Ed Norton was in character. Art tripled Jackie. He was the sympathetic character. I don't think Jackie would have made it as Ralph Kramden without Art as Ed Norton. Years later when CBS offered Gleason a new variety show, he wouldn't go back without Art. Gleason understood talent and character. Audrey Meadows was their safety net. She connected them to reality by reeling them in when they went out too far.

Once you created a person or characters the audience could believe in, you were on your way. If you point to any one of my writers, their comedic legacies are bound up with the characters they created. Carl Reiner and Rob and Laura Petrie. Mel Brooks and Maxwell Smart. Max Bialystock and Leo Bloom. Larry Gelbart and Hawkeye Pierce, and Trapper John McIntyre. Aaron Ruben and Andy Taylor and Barney Fife. Joe Stein and Tevye the Milkman. Mike Stewart and Conrad Birdie and Dolly Levi. Mel Tolkin and Archie and Edith Bunker. Neil Simon and Felix Unger and Oscar Madison. Woody Allen and Alvy Singer. All are enduring characters that are fundamentally believable as people, which enables them to be tremendously funny characters as well.

In Britain, the same thing happened. *Monty Python's Flying Circus*, for example, is one of the best things to come out of there because it gives you an understanding of the British character and what they're doing. *Monty Python* made fun of the British character. We made fun of the American character.

A sketch could begin with something as simple as trying to wipe a spot off a lapel at a party. Carl comes in and says to me, "Gee, that's a lovely jacket." And then he says, "There's a spot on your lapel. Let me try and get it out. It'll take a second." He tries to brush it away with two fingers. Then he starts to really brush it. He takes a fingernail and starts to scrape it. Then come the liquids: "Maybe a little water, a little club soda, maybe a little milk, it has calcium." No, that doesn't work. "Maybe a little benzene will do the trick." None of these remedies are getting the spot out. They're actually having the opposite effect, making it larger. "Why don't I take the jacket off and wash it" is Carl's next suggestion. He uses a washboard and basin. As he is going through all these machinations, I'm just watching it all happen. "Maybe a little fire will take it out," he says. This goes on for five or six minutes, and at the end of the sketch all Carl has succeeded in doing is destroying my jacket. I look at him, and I slowly take two fingers and start wiping a stain off of his jacket. I say, "Maybe a little fire will take this out." It's all in the timing.

The writers all thought I was a Stradivarius and they were the collective Mozarts writing the music for it. The Stradivarius adds to the color of the music, it adds to the tone, and makes you feel you can do anything you want, so I understood their feeling.

I always thought of the writers as the violins. As an instrument, the violin is true and you depend on that. There are violins and there are violins, and then there are the masterpieces, Stradivarius, Guarnerius, and a few others whose names escape me. They were not only made out of the finest woods, the right glue and the right varnish, but by trained and passionate craftsmen with the finest hearts. You can get a violin in a pawnshop for five bucks and you can get a violin that is custom made, and then there are the masterpieces that sell for $5 million. And you depend on the tones coming out of the great violins that you wouldn't get from the ordinary ones. That's where great music comes from. And you always have to live up to your instrument.

Sometimes a writer would stand up and say something and it would be funny, but I would say it's not funny for me. It's not just about whether people will laugh. You have to make up your mind because you're going to have to really play it. The performer has to convince himself that what he is doing is real and true before he can convince the audience.

On the other hand, I would take things in the scripts and often go beyond them. I was constantly testing how much the comedic traffic would bear. Will the audience be with me? If the audience is with you, you take flight because things come to you.

A good example of how a sketch was created and the pace with which it evolved was something we did called "Six Tickets." The idea started with the usual phrase from one of the writers: "I got it, Sid! I'm working in the office, the boss comes in and says 'Bob?' I jump up, 'Yes, sir?' 'We have some executives coming in from out of town and we bought them six tickets to the big opening night show of 'Snap Your Garter.' They can't make it, so I'm giving you the six tickets and you can see it tonight.' 'Oh, gee, I've heard of it. That's a big show.' 'But Bob, it's formal. You have to wear a tuxedo.' "

I liked that idea, partly because it meant I had to call my wife. We had just learned of a new technological innovation called the split screen. "You mean you could have two people from two places on the same screen at the same time?" I asked. "You mean you wouldn't have to cut back and forth in a telephone conversation?" To comedy writers it was as significant a breakthrough as splitting the atom. It was as if we were in a cave and had just discovered fire.

This was a perfect tool for the sketch. I've got to call my wife, my wife has to call the other girls, the other girls have to call their husbands. Before then we couldn't have shown all of that activity. By putting a board in on the side of the split screen, we divided the screen three ways to display three of the conversations simultaneously: "We have to wear tuxedos, so bring down my tuxedo . . . my cuff links are in the aspirin box . . . give me the number of the ticket and I'll pick up your stole from storage . . . And you call him and he'll call you and you've got all these people . . ."

I say we'll all meet at the Crying Owl Bar and we'll have some drinks and hors d'oeuvres there and then we'll go to the Spinning Web, where we'll have a nice dinner. And then we'll go to the Dinot Hotel where we'll change into tuxedos and dresses. And from there we'll get a cab and we'll all go to the theater. That, at least, was the original plan.

We started to get deeper into the crafting of the sketch, filling in the details. After work, we'll meet at the Crying Owl Bar; we come in one at a time. "Is there anybody here who's going to see a show tonight? Did you see a guy with black hair — he was here but he said he was going to the hotel." And meanwhile we decided it had to be raining that night.

Every aspect of the plan unravels; everything starts to go wrong. We all met at the restaurant, dripping wet from the rain, but we couldn't get a reservation. So we said let's go to the hotel, at least we can have a bite there. We'll dry off and put on new clothes. We get to the hotel, and the World Series is in town. There are no rooms. "You haven't got a room? Holy cow! What are we gonna do now?"

The girls are all dressed, so the men have to change into tuxedos without a hotel room to do it in. We go to the theater, where everybody else is in tuxedos, and what do you know, there are three telephone booths! We go into the telephone booths and try to change there. I've got Howie's clothes on, Howie has Carl's clothes, and Carl has my clothes, and we're trading pants from one booth to another.

Small details were significant in the

development of a sketch and helped determine whether the audience would follow us. In The Commuters sketch entitled "Seven Dwarfs Bet," Carl bets me $100 that I'm wrong about the names of the Seven Dwarfs. The writers, who could argue for hours over which numbers were funny and which weren't, deliberated over how much to set the bet at. In those days, $100 got your attention. For my character, that was a big bet. It was important money. A thousand dollars would've been too outrageous; $50 would have been too little. My character ended up putting in a call to Walt Disney himself in Los Angeles. "Hello, Mr. Disney," I say in a deep, self-important voice, "this is Bob Victor calling from New York City. *Long distance.* Do you know the names of the seven dwarfs?" Even he doesn't know. I drop back to my regular voice. "Well, does your wife know?" I ask. "When your kid wakes up, call me. Just reverse the charges."

We could build a sketch out of the smallest thing that happened in life, like who was going to pick up the check at a restaurant: "No, no, no — I'm picking it up. Oh no, no. I'll pick up the check — okay, well, I'll toss you for it . . . No, there will not be tossing, I'm taking the check, this is my dinner . . . But I asked you and you accepted." The argument almost escalates into a brawl. And then the wives start to argue. You get the idea.

One time we thought smaller still and came up with the idea that I could be a fly that wakes up on the ceiling of a suburban home. He washes his six legs, stretches, and then flies down under the toaster. To his shock, it's clean; there are no crumbs anywhere. "Well, maybe in the sink. No crumbs. Oh, that's it — the maid was here yesterday. I'll have to go fly downtown for breakfast . . . Where's the hole in the screen?"

He gets this leg out, this leg, then that leg, and then another leg. "Where's downtown?" A little sniff. "Oh yes, it's that way . . . Oh, hello, Mr. Caterpillar. You're putting your shoes on; you've got all those legs, it'll take all morning. Hey, Harry how are you? I haven't seen you in a little while. What's been going on with you?

"Oh you got married. A couple of weeks ago. You had the reception at Garbage Dump 2. That's a gourmet place where they have the class food. That's where they dump the stuff from the Stork Club and Lindy's. Any children? Three and a half million? Wow! All of them girls. And not one of them writes. Well, so long Harry. I'm going to have breakfast.

"I ate at that restaurant the other day. Oh a Greek restaurant. Look at that feta cheese. Acres and acres of cheese, and it's all mine. Oh, look out, a guy with a newspaper. Oh, he's really out to swat me today."

I get out of his way. Now I am stuck. I fell for the oldest trick in the book: flypaper.

"Hey, Harry, it's a good thing you came to this restaurant. Can you help me out of this? Don't touch anything. It's sticky. Just pull on my legs. Thanks, pal. I'll never forget you. I think I'll fly home now. Will you look at that sign: DDT KILLS FLIES IN- STANTLY. Boy, there's a lot of hate in this world."

Sometimes great one-liners can result from unhappy situations. For example, Carl and I played the fathers of two fighting eight-year-old boys who are called into the principal's office. "I used to get beat up by a bully in grade school," I tell Carl. "In high school we actually became friends. And today, that bully is my wife." Priceless.

As we were building and evolving our sketch comedy, we would look for new types of sketches that had legs (not cater- pillar legs). We liked the idea of recurring characters and themes. It gave us something we could start with and something the audience could connect with. During *Your Show of Shows*, we came up with what we called cliché sketches. The cliché sketches were inspired by Imogene. She sounded like she came from the Midwest and always spoke in clichés. So we began to develop satires of clichés and platitudes. They were all typical conversations that people would have. We played parents talking about taking their children to school for the first time, two superstitious people pretending not to be superstitious, or two strangers who meet while talking in line outside a movie theater. We played parents discussing the psychology of raising children in modern times: "I think the old method of spanking a child is passé," Immy tells me. "I say don't just spank a child," I reply. "Talk to the child, reason with him, and find out what's on his mind. And then when you find out the reason, the real cause — *then* belt him."

We were two parents at a high school graduation:

Coca: There's my daughter . . . fourth from the right.
Sid: Oh, I see her. The redhead with the

plunging neckline and the high heels.

Coca: It's a stage she's going through. In a couple of weeks, she'll be back to her natural brown hair. Where's your son?

Sid: He's the one standing right next to your daughter with his mouth open.

There was the cliché wedding:

Coca: You know how they met, it was so romantic. He was picking up the garbage. At that moment he fell in love with her.

Sid: Did you hear, her father is opening a store for him.

Coca: You think she's that beautiful?

Sid: With a store, she's beautiful enough.

And then there was a simple conversation about a dog:

Sid: I like a playful dog. I once had a Great Dane. They're so playful and affectionate, you know. Whenever he'd see me, he'd jump up and knock me down, tear my clothes, and drag me all over the living room floor . . . I was afraid to go home.

Coca: Dogs are really faithful. We had a neighbor of ours who treated his dog miserably . . . never fed him on time. Well, one day he just up and left. The dog didn't leave that front porch. He was faithful. He would never leave. Well, about two years later, the master returned. The dog just stood there, watching his master come down the path and onto the porch. And when that dog saw his owner, his ears went up and he started to smell his master.

Sid: And then what happened?

Coca: That dog ripped him to pieces.

A funny conversation can develop from anywhere. This one started with nothing more than two ordinary guys, truck drivers on the road, and then spiraled beautifully out of control.

Carl: Boy, I'll sure be glad when this trip is over. I'm gonna hit the sack and sleep for forty-eight hours.

Sid: Not me.

Carl: Why, what're you gonna do?

Sid: I'm gonna take a bath, a shave and I'm going out on a date.

Carl: A date? Boy, I don't know a girl that beautiful I'd wanna take her out after this trip . . . Who are you taking out?

Sid: Peggy.

Carl: Peggy.

Sid: What?

Carl: Nothing. It's just that she's too

beautiful for you. She's a very pretty girl, and she can get any romantic guy she wants to.

Sid: Wait a minute. Are you suggesting that I'm not romantic?

Carl: Yeah.

Sid: I'm just as romantic as the next guy, and maybe even romantic-er. And when I get all dressed up in a suit and white gloves I'm beautiful.

Carl: What you're trying to say is that you feel that you are romantic enough to get Peggy to marry you.

Sid: If I wanted to, yeah.

Carl: (Laughs) You're just interested in her cause she's pretty.

Sid: I'm not marrying Peggy just because she's pretty. I'm marrying her because we got things in common.

Carl: Like what?

Sid: Handball . . . We play every Sunday morning. And I respect her. She's got a beautiful left hand.

Carl: Don't give me that. You'd marry any girl with a pretty face.

Sid: I would not.

Carl: No? You mean to tell me if a girl like Marilyn Monroe asked you to marry her you wouldn't marry her?

Sid: No.

Carl: You're kidding. You wouldn't marry Marilyn Monroe?

Sid: No.

Carl: If she begged you?

Sid: No.

Carl: You know who I'm talking about — the movie star . . . Marilyn Monroe.

Sid: Yeah, I know, I know. The answer is still no.

Carl: Every man in the world would give his eyeteeth to marry Marilyn Monroe.

Sid: Let 'em! I don't wanna marry her!

Carl: Do you know what you're saying? Marilyn Monroe? The most beautiful girl in the world, and you don't wanna marry her?

Sid: Look, once and for all, I refuse to marry Marilyn Monroe, and don't try to keep pushing her off on me!

Carl: How about Lana Turner?

Sid: Look, I thought I made it very clear to you yesterday I'm not marrying Lana Turner. And don't start with Hedy Lamarr again.

Carl: All right.

Sid: Lemme put it this way. Now if you was a girl like Peggy and knowing me and my emotions, would you marry me?

Carl: Stanley, should I give it to you straight?

Sid: Yeah.

Carl: No, I wouldn't marry you.

Sid: Why?

Carl: Because I'm not in love with you.

Sid: What?

Carl: Oh, I'm very fond of you but I don't love you enough to marry you. But I don't wanna marry the first truck driver that asks me. I'm young yet. I wanna look around. If I was Peggy. You understand, don't you?

Sid: Sure, Charlie. I appreciate your frankness. Get outta the truck!

Carl: What're you getting sore about. Just cause I wouldn't marry you.

Sid: Look, if I was Peggy and we've been friends for seven years, I'd marry you.

Carl: That's because I'm more romantic than you.

Sid: Another ten miles and we're there.

Carl: What're you stopping for?

Sid: Did you see what I saw?

Carl: What?

Sid: There's a bride standing there in the road.

Carl: A what?

Sid: A bride . . . bride!

Carl: You mean a bride . . . in a wedding gown?

Sid: That's right.

Carl: Is she carrying a bouquet of flowers?

Sid: Yeah, yeah . . .

Carl: White satin shoes?

Sid: Yeah, a bride!!

Carl: Stanley, you better let me drive.

Sid: Look, I'm telling you. I just saw a bride in the road . . .

Carl: Hey, you're right. What's a bride doing in the middle of a highway in the dead of night?

Sid: I don't know. Maybe she's on her honeymoon.

Carl: Honeymoon alone? Where's her spouse?

Sid: Maybe they couldn't afford to go together . . . So they just sent her.

Carl: Ah that's crazy!

Sid: Maybe she's in dire straits. Let's give her a lift.

Carl: Okay. Wait a minute. You know the company rule. No riders.

Sid: Yeah, but look at her standing there. She's crying. Let's pick her up.

Carl: It might mean our jobs if we get caught, like if they found a clue, like if they found rice in the cab.

Sid: We could say we were eating Chinese food. Let's pick her up.

Carl: Okay.

Sid: I beg your pardon, Miss. We couldn't help but notice you in your bridal gown. Can we give you a lift to Niagara Falls? Swell. Go on, Charlie . . . Help her up . . . Take her bouquet.

Carl: Okay lady, here let me help you.

Howie: All right, you guys, this is a stickup. (Takes their money and goes) All right, on your way.

Sid: Close the door, Charlie. I read about this guy in the morning paper. The Bandit Bride.

Carl: And you had to stop and give him a lift . . . the poor, poor bride.

Sid: Aaaaaa, shut up!!!

Working chefs and waiters were always a viable theme. I love food. Because I grew up in the restaurant business, I always associated food with family, and I always tried to put food in the sketches because people know it's a comforting feeling. I also love watching people eat. You can learn a lot about people by the way they eat. We tried to show how differently people eat, and how people eat when they're mad — sometimes they just dabble and sometimes they wolf it down. Food says a lot about how you treat people, as well.

In a sketch set at a posh, high-class French restaurant, I was Pierre the headwaiter. Everything was done with flair.

"Missuer, your soufflé will be out shortly." Except every time the door to the kitchen would swing open, flames would shoot out. The kitchen was on fire, but I downplayed it. We continued business as usual throughout the fire as if nothing happened. "I presume you want the soufflé hot? Henri! Two soufflés hot," I yell. "Don't worry, Missuer Pierre, it'll be hot," is the off camera response. All hell is breaking loose, and firemen are running around with hoses. I do not lose my composure. "We are just cooling off your soufflé," I tell the customer. Someone ordered Jell-O, and they got it with a soup spoon because it had turned to water. "Would you like a cigar, Missuer. You can light it up as you pass the kitchen on your way out." We even gave the patrons change for their checks with singed money.

A circus skit we did, "Caesaro's Flip-Flop Circus," also made comedy out of make-believe misfortune. It starts with circus performers doing elaborate acrobatic tricks and moves. Carl, Howie, and I come out in tights and leotards and twirl napkins with the same labored expressions as the serious acrobats.

Another group of performers come out, including a unicyclist juggling hula hoops while a leggy woman does cartwheels around him and collects the hoops. The three of us come out again with a foot-high three-legged stool. We take turns jumping over the stool. I sit down and it looks like my two colleagues are going to lift me up, when I jump up and the three of us miraculously lift the two-pound stool together. Let me tell you, there's nothing easy about the circus life.

The clowns and the showgirls come out once again and do flips and cartwheels. The three of us return with three chairs. As the audience waits to see what we'll do, three showgirls sit down in the chairs. We grab their wrists, strain for a few moments, and then lean in and kiss the girls.

A juggler comes out with three pins and we come out again, each holding three pins. But we put them at our feet and kick them off to the side. Finally, we put a beautiful woman in a cannon, and Carl and Howie move out and prepare to catch her. The cannon fires and there is no woman to be caught. We look inside the barrel of the cannon and make a sad face. Always the gentleman, I turn the opening of the barrel away.

Some sketches could get a little more violent than others. In "Which Way to

Riverdale?" Howie innocently asks Imogene and me for directions at the bus station. Imogene and I begin to argue over whether Howie should grab the number 5 or number 7 bus. We are each emphatic about our positions. As the argument escalates, we grab Howie, rip his clothes off, and destroy his suitcase. Imogene is hugging and kissing him, flipping him upside down. There were many times where Howie did not get through a sketch with most of his clothes intact. We made sure he always had underwear on.

Although there was a decidedly physical component to it, our comedy wasn't slapstick. We didn't throw pies around, and it wasn't vaudeville shpritz humor. And even when our humor seemed topical, it didn't have an expiration date on it, which is one of the reasons it is still funny today. In one sketch I played the CEO of a corporation on a train en route to Denver, reviewing a report with a nosy old woman sitting next to me.

Old Woman: Oh the Denver Amalgamated Company.
Sid: I am the CEO. You know us?
Old Woman: Oh yes. I own stock in the company. I think you're all a bunch of crooks!

That same 1955 interchange could have

easily taken place in 2003 with an executive of Enron, Worldcom, or one of another dozen companies. Some things never change.

Another sketch had to do with one of the fixtures of 1950s television, the quiz show. People loved to see other people squirm on television. They do now more than ever, with all the reality shows out there. When I was a little kid, something called *The Sixty-Four Dollar Question* was very popular on the radio. Now sixty-four dollars could barely get you to the studio and back home.

Even though the shows were popular, it was a time when the questions were serious and complicated. You had to know art, history, science, and politics, without multiple-choice questions, help from the audience, or lifelines.

Before the scandals that ended the quiz shows, we did a sketch called "Break Your Brains." Carl played a synthesis of all game show hosts as he announced the return of last week's contestants: "Ronald Gordon, an eight-year-old nuclear scientist and expert on comic books; Mrs. Marjorie Barnes, a ninety-three-year-old grandmother from St. Louis, Missouri, whose category is pole vaulting; and Rudolph Schmidt, a baker from Wysetta, Minnesota, whose category is bakeries in Wysetta, Minnesota."

I played Harry Hempstead, a nervous, returning twenty-five-week champion whose topic was "anything." I am exhausted from my long reign, hugging on Carl's shoulder and crying "no more, no more."

Shaking hands with each competitor, I said, "Good evening. How are you, I hope you all lose." No one at the time would have said anything like that. Now nasty competition is de rigueur for game shows.

I compose myself and we prepare to begin the quiz. Carl asks how being on the show has affected my life. I answer, "It's been a wonderful experience. I've had my picture in the newspaper. I've been interviewed on the radio. And was beaten up once and robbed twice."

I had already won a quarter of a million dollars. The joke was, should I keep it, or should I risk it to win the same quarter million. "You have everything to lose and nothing to win," Carl says. "Would you rather take it home or would you rather go for the same quarter million dollars?" I am offered the choice of accepting the money as a college fund for my children or as $250,000 in matched luggage.

We used a clip from *The War of the Worlds*

with Raymond Massey and Sir Cedric Hardwicke that showed the elaborate and fanciful construction of a city to simulate the crafting of the question on a card, which popped out of a computer. We knew how to rehearse the props so we wouldn't be surprised by anything.

While this is happening, I am sweating in the "humiliation booth" (I spent a lot of time trapped in booths during my years on television). The show's advertiser was Poopatrol. At the time, the sponsor's name would be plastered all over the microphones, the booths, and every other free spot on the set, so we did the same.

They play an aria and ask me to identify it. While I am thinking, they blast another piece of music.

Carl now asks me a number of questions, very quickly, "From what opera is 'Caranomi' taken? Name the five tenors who sang the leading role before 1930. Name the opera companies for which these tenors sang. In which opera companies were these operas performed and name at least four out of the five leading ladies that sang in these roles with these tenors. Name at least five of his unpublished operas. Name his wife and the first names of his children. You have fifteen seconds to answer these questions. Take every minute of those fifteen seconds!"

They blast yet another piece of frenetic music.

Carl asks, "Okay, Harry, what are your answers?"

" 'Caranomi' is from *Rigoletto*. It was first sung by Enrico Caruso then sung by Freddy Peliche Chalicio, then sung by Genito Bellini Caruso Calicasso Salvani, Micaloso Calvini Jampierst, Tony Galenti, Tommy Direnzo. It was first performed at the Metropolitan Opera Company, the Chicago Opera Company, the St. Louis Biz Opera Company, the St. Paul Muni Opera Company, The Role Opera Company. It was performed February 18, 1801, 1803, 1804, the Red Wing Theater, 1755, 1836, 1844, 1906, 1945. The leading ladies were Luisa Teresa, Marisa Teresa, Maria Angelo, Dolores del Rio, Moris Laya, Bess Myerson. It was written by Verdi, his unpublished works are *Corinna de la Mora*, *The Nina*, *The Pinta*, and *The Santa Maria*, *The Christa de Foro* (lots of Italian doubletalk) and *The Girl from the Golden West!*"

Carl responds: "It's absolutely phenomenal, it's amazing. Absolutely every answer was wrong! But in answering your questions you used two hundred and fifty seconds, which at a thousand dollars a second is $250,000." He counts out three bills and pays me in cash.

Carl was able to showcase a lot of his comedic skills as the host of the quiz show. It was a real virtuoso piece for him.

Funny as "Break Your Brains" was, if I were producing today, this would be the kind of sketch I would cut down. I would take down the advertisements and the girls coming in and out. In the era of the remote control and more limited attention spans, I don't think it would hold the attention of the audience as easily.

During the dress rehearsals of *Caesar's Hour*, Milt Kamen would take my place on the set, and I went into the control room to help the technical crew direct the shots. Comedy is very intricate. There are very few people who can shoot comedy well. You've got to know where the laugh is supposed to be. The normal inclination for a director is to follow the person speaking. In comedy when you see a character starting to talk, you have to follow the person who is listening and reacting to what is being said. The laugh isn't always with the person who says it. It's the reaction. "But we need to keep the camera on the guy who is talking." "No you don't," I would tell the editors. "You follow the laugh." That's why it's so important for actors to listen and not just wait for their cue. When editors get in there, they generally know nothing about comedy. They know time. "I gotta get it down to this time." So they chop. Too often they don't know what they're chopping.

There is a saying that "Comedy is a man in trouble." I often found you could take even very serious subjects and work them for both comedy and pathos. For instance: There's a rich man standing on a deck of an oceangoing yacht, smoking a cigar. And there's another guy in a rowboat, fishing. All of a sudden the yacht comes bearing down on the rowboat, like an ocean liner at top speed. And the rich guy's standing there smoking his cigar, while the guy in the rowboat is trying frantically to get out of the way. The bow wave from the wake of the yacht throws the rowboat over, and the rich man does not even notice. Who are you going to follow, the man on the yacht smoking the cigar or the man whose rowboat has just been overturned? Naturally, the rowboat, no question about it. You know that the man on the yacht is going to finish the cigar and go to bed. The audience will stay with the guy who's in trouble because everyone knows what trouble is. You know he's not going to drown. You can see him climb back into the rowboat and get home, so you know you don't have to worry about him. You can just relax and laugh.

To show you how drama slips into comedy, I had an idea for a sketch that we never did. It starts with an old married couple sitting in the parlor on rocking chairs, reading the paper. There's a flag in the window with two stars. All of a sudden there's a knock on the door. A telegram is delivered. The wife opens the telegram and reads it. It is from the Defense Department: "Sorry to tell you that your son has been killed." The wife starts to cry. She leaves the parlor to go upstairs, but she faints on the staircase. The husband reads the telegram and then goes after his wife. He tries to help her up, but he trips on the second step and falls down as well. They're both just lying there. Then a dog runs in from the street and starts barking, and people are coming in, curious and concerned, asking, "What's going on?" They see the couple lying on the stairs. And they all start to help. "You pick her up. No, pick him up first. Get his legs. Put her head up and cross her arms and take her off his head, and watch out. No, don't hold her up, slide her underneath, hold him straight. If you're gonna push, push him under . . ." All of a sudden, this tragic situation becomes a comedy. Trying to save the couple, the friends and neighbors start hurting them more. The routine starts to get funny. Because when you go too far in a serious mode, it inevitably slips into comedy. When drama is overacted or overwritten, humor is what results.

That example is an extreme version of the connection between comedy and pathos. You cannot show someone killed, at least not that way. It's not funny. A concept like that may work in an experimental theater setting. It worked on *M*A*S*H* because it was set during wartime. The audience was attuned to it and willing to accept it. But it would be dangerous for something like *Your Show of Shows* and *Caesar's Hour* because it would be hard to tell how the audience would take it.

One of the funniest lines we ever had was in "The Coward," a silent movie satire set during the Civil War. Naturally I played the coward. The scene opens in a recruiting station. Two guys go in first and I'm next on line. I put down a note. "This is from my mother," I tell the recruiting officer. It said, "Please excuse Howard from the Civil War as he has a cold." It still makes me laugh.

It was a ridiculous premise, but it was part of a more elaborate plot. I didn't want to go to war, and the audience connected with that. Then the Southerners came up from Gettysburg and I saw them in my house and now I have to fight to save my wife and children. It was a sketch about the Civil War, and at the same time it wasn't. There was a larger theme. It was showing what people do when faced with fear and change.

That's the kind of work we did. The audience understood both the comedy and the underlying message. They understood what I was talking about. Nobody is that brave that he would volunteer for death in the abstract. You're not fighting for just the United States. You're fighting for this guy, right next to you, and he's fighting for you. You can bet your life on that. And in a comedic context, being scared is okay.

When you think about it, laughter and crying are the same emotion. They are two sides of the same coin. When you cry too much you start to laugh; you get hysterical. When you laugh too much you start to cry. Tears come to your eyes. They're both releases. There's no such thing as a monopole, there's nothing that just goes around a north pole or a south pole. That's the center of comedy. That and belief.

I believed, and still do, that you take sketch comedy as seriously as you would if you were performing Shakespeare. If you try and act funny, it won't be funny. If you act naturally and let the situation make you funny, then you can build on that. Once you get the audience going, then you can do anything else, because you have the audience laughing and you control it. When someone doesn't know whether to laugh or cry, your comedy is working.

Chapter 10

THE PROFESSOR

Of all the recurring characters I've played, the Professor is probably the one I am remembered for most. The man claims to be an expert on everything, but he's a bluff; he really knows nothing. His saving grace is seeing him get out of the situations he gets himself into. While he's saying, "You'll pardon me for laughing on you," we're laughing at him.

Part of the inspiration for the Professor came from Jack Pearl, a comedian I met while I was on Broadway with *Make Mine Manhattan*. A very warm man and a very talented comedian, Jack was best known for playing Baron Munchhausen on the radio in the 1930s. They called him the "Great Bluffer." He would tell a crazy, unbelievable story and when he was challenged about its truthfulness he'd snap back: "Vas you dere, Sharlie?" Before Jack was done, he'd made that expression a household phrase.

The Professor was a long time developing. We started with a recurring sketch called "Nonentities in the News" that was set at LaGuardia Airport because we figured an airport was a good place to find arriving eccentrics. A reporter in a trench coat would interview a strange character who had just gotten off a plane. I was always the Deplaning Strange Character, a role that had me playing everyone from Jungle Boy to Dr. Spaghetti, who didn't hesitate to tell the audience how to cook and eat various forms of pasta, and what to eat it with. "Let the ice cream melt fast as the spaghetti gets al dente. You get the main course and the dessert together. It saves time." The original idea was that I would play a different nationality each week, first a Frenchman, then a German, and then an Italian, all within the same interview format.

One week, I called Eve's Costumes, a big vaudeville supply house in New York City. They catered to Broadway shows, vaudeville houses, nightclubs, and similar productions. They had some very talented people. I told them that I was going to play a European professor whose dress was immaculately sloppy. They sent over a complete costume, just like that: the swallowtail coat, the flattened top hat and wide tie, the yellow W. C. Fields vest with the roll collar, and the baggy striped pants with the suspenders.

It was a very rich, broken-down looking outfit, and it stayed that way until I donated it to the Smithsonian Institution fifteen years ago. I put it on, mussed up my hair on the sides, looked in the mirror and said, "This is a German professor. Hello, herr doctor." And that was it. With Carl Reiner as the imperturbable interviewer never without a trench coat and a notepad, the Professor sketches got progressively better.

Reporter: Hello there, this is your roving reporter, Carl Reiner, here at LaGuardia Airport, awaiting the arrival of a planeload of eminent visitors, among them the distinguished Viennese authority on mountain climbing and one of the greatest guides in the world. His new book on mountain climbing has just been published. It's called "What Do You Need It For?" Please welcome Professor Gut von Fraidykat.

Reporter: Professor, you seem in good spirits today.

Professor: Well, I just conquered Mount Richtvichtrichtigrechtziglauden. I conquered it! But my partner is still dangling. He climbed it with roller skates. I told him not to do it. But he insisted. He was a sweet fella. He was on the other end of this rope, and all of a sudden, nothing! But you can't let your spirits get down.

Reporter: I see. Well, Professor, I imagine you wear that rope about you in memory and respect for him.

Professor: No, it keeps my pants up.

Reporter: Professor, who do you consider the best mountain climber of them all?

Professor: Jim Richardson!

Reporter: Jim Richardson?

Professor: He could scramble over a mountain. Do you know Mount Dingdallen? Dis fella could climb a mountain. He went up that mountain in three days, fourteen hours, and seven minutes.

Reporter: Is that a record, Professor?

Professor: No, he broke the record on the vay down. Ten seconds, flat! Flat! He broke the record, he broke his head, everything!

Reporter: What is the most dangerous mountain in the whole world?

Professor: Mount Slippery. In the Slippery Valley. Big, foreboding. It's sheer cliffs.

Reporter: What can one do in an emergency? When the rope breaks?

Professor: You didn't read that chapter, on emergencies?

Reporter: No.

Professor: When you are on the side of the mountain and your rope breaks, you have two seconds to act. The first thing you do is you start to scream, and you keep screaming all the vay down.

Reporter: Why would you do that?

Professor: So they'll know where to find you.

Reporter: Is there another alternative?

Professor: There's another alternative, when you see your rope breaks, you have two seconds again, you can spread your arms and you start to fly as hard as you can.

Reporter: But Professor, humans can't fly.

Professor: How do you know, you may be the first one, buddy. Fly, fly! You could always go back to screaming. That's always working for you!

Reporter: I hate to bring this up, but your friend Hans Goodfellow, was he a screamer or a flyer?

Professor: He was a flying screamer! And a big crasher. He bounced a lot too. A crasher and a bouncer.

Reporter: Professor, have you ever fallen from any heights?

Professor: You're looking at a kid that took a flop. Pikes Peak. I took a flop from there, seven thousand six hundred and forty two feet.

Reporter: Did you hurt yourself badly?
Professor: See that? (Points to pinky finger) That's all that's left of the original me. Everything else is new! I had a great surgeon. I used to be a short redhead.

Because there were so many things you could pretend to be an authority about, the Professor had no trouble becoming a recurring character. As Professor Ludwig von Spacebrain, for instance, he was an expert on jet propulsion, insisting that "the most important problem in space today is, I would say, closet space."

Then there was Professor Hookline von Sinker, the world's greatest fisherman, who lost a tussle with a can of sardines (he couldn't get it open) and recounted an epic battle with a silver shark that lasted for over four months. The only reason he finally let go was because it was the end of the fishing season.

One of my favorites was Professor Ludwig von Fossil, one hell of an archeologist.

Reporter: What was the greatest discovery you've made as an excavator and archeologist?
Professor: You know, the greatest secret in archeology is the Secret of Titten-Tottens Tomb and I decided to make it my lifework.

After many years, I found the Secret of Titten-Tottens Tomb.

Reporter: What was it, Doctor?

Professor: You think I'm gonna tell you? You got another guess coming. You take that trip.

Reporter: Professor, what is the most revolutionary discovery you made in all of your travels?

Professor: I found an old civilization. It was a matriarchal society where the women were the important people — the men were nothing. The women were the rulers. They were the heads of the government. They were in charge of everything.

Reporter: Where was this, Doctor?

Professor: In Cincinnati.

The Professor was still alive and well when we made the transition to *Caesar's Hour*. He was a character that had legs as well as an accent. He became a regular on our recurring satire of the superserious talk show *Omnibus*, hosted by Alistair Cooke, which we turned into "Ominous" with Carl as Aristotle Cookie.

On one show, Aristotle introduced the Professor as "one of the leading authorities on happiness and an expert on marriage. His two books are *My Twenty Years of Marriage* and *Great Battles of History*. Professor Ludwig von Henpecked."

"I love you darling," I said to my wife, putting my face up to the camera, "but you don't put starch in a T-shirt." I then began to expound on married life.

"The origin of marriage started in the cave. Woman was someone who came in to clean once a week for a dollar and a half and carfare. Man gets the idea, why should I pay a woman to clean. I can marry her and she can do the cleaning and the ironing for free. And that was the beginning of the Iron Age."

"Professor, what is the force that pushes people together to get married?" Aristotle asks.

"The girl's mother. She forces the marriage all the time. She cooks the meal and says, 'My daughter made that.' "

"How do you feel about marrying for money?"

"That's a loaded question. If the girl is loaded, it's no question!"

The Professor became such a strong character that we confidently turned him loose, letting him leave the airport and "Ominous" and confound people where they worked and played.

The Professor advised the board of

directors of struggling Mammoth Pictures on a new musical:

Professor: I'll tell you what we do. Get Beethoven. Ludwig is not only a great composer, but he's also a good guy.
Executive: Professor, Beethoven's dead.
Professor: Beethoven's gone? Ludwig gone? You don't pick up a paper for a few days . . . I'll tell you what we do. Call Mozart.
Executive: Professor, Mozart is also dead.
Professor: Wolfgang is gone? I'm sick from that. I was so close with him. What was it, an accident? They were both in the same bus or something? Beethoven and Mozart, verklumpt. The world is upside down. All right, I'll tell you what we do. We get Tchaikovsky.
Executive: Tchaikovsky is dead.
Professor: That's where I got you, Sparky. I just made that name up. There is no Tchaikovsky!

The Professor also turned up to address a convention of the United Society of Amateur Magicians as Professor Houdini von Hoffmeyer, the master of prestidigitation, legerdemain, and illusion.

I use a box the size of a closet to try and make a chorus girl disappear. We close the doors and the girl doesn't disappear. "Did you tell the agency I wanted a girl that disappears?" I close the door again and two girls appear. Then three. Then Howie Morris as my son, complete with ridiculous-looking lederhosen, is transported from Europe. Then five girls appear. I get in the box with them, and the girls start screaming. I open the door, stick my head out, and ask Carl, "Can you get me some ginger ale and ice?" The Professor was always ready to party.

In another sketch, Carl and Howie played scientists working on the XXM4, a space rocket. They're so desperate they enlist the services of Professor Ludwig von Vacuum.

Professor: Anything for science.
Carl: The XXM4. Will it fly?
Professor: No. But it's a nice Christmas item. (Throws it on the floor). It didn't fly — it didn't even bounce.
Carl: How did you prepare against lack of gravity?
Professor: For seven months I slept in a washing machine.
Carl: We would like you to test the pressure tester. So far we have only used monkeys.
Professor: No! You keep going with the monkeys. I don't vant to put monkeys out of work.

They put me in the pressure tester,

which looked a lot like a booth on *The $64,000 Question*. "Could I have an expert in there with me?" I ask. "The marine had an expert in there with him. All he answered were questions on soup and how to make wine." At 100,000 feet of pressure, I have a headache and I think my nose will explode. At 150,000 feet of pressure, they tell me I can now go to Mars. "You can go to Mars," I tell them, getting out of the pressure tester. "I'm going home and sleeping in the washing machine."

The Professor got so celebrated he started to have an impact on the real world. At least that's what Mike Wallace once said.

In the '50s, long before *60 Minutes*, Mike did a show on Channel 5, a local New York station, called *Night Beat*. Mike would chain-smoke while he grilled the guests and ask very sharp, probing questions. Invariably, beads of sweat would form on foreheads as Mike went in for the kill. So we did a parody with Carl playing Mike and the Professor as his latest victim.

Reporter: Let us meet Professor Ludwig von Integrity.
Professor: Don't start schtooking me right away with the tough questions, you know

what I mean. Ask some easy questions, like what size shoes I take, you know.

Reporter: Yes, Professor.

Professor: But don't give the schtook away.

Reporter: There's a picture of you in 1923, Professor? Is that you with your arm around a chorus girl?

Professor: You start right away with the schtook. I was just passing by and they needed a picture. And she put her arm around me. You can't stop that. But . . .

Reporter: And you are supposed to have sold over $450,000 dollars worth of stock.

Professor: Yes. Tinsel stock.

Reporter: You say you weren't fixing a fight? You haven't said what you did with the gold mine.

Professor: You only talk schtooks. I noticed that from the first question. Why do you keep schtooking into everything?

Reporter: Your 1935 income tax bill . . .

Professor: Oh . . .

While I was being interrogated, the camera cut to my face in a very tight shot, just in mid-forehead. Perspiration was dropping down my face, off my nose, and my eyes. There was a guy behind me with a big sponge just out of camera range, slowly squeezing it so water dripped down my face in a torrent of sweat. The Professor was a little nervous.

According to Mike, this was around the time he was negotiating with ABC for his show to be nationally syndicated. The way he tells the story, they sat down one afternoon to negotiate a contract with the network, and the negotiations weren't going very well. Everyone took a break that night to watch *Caesar's Hour*, which just happened to be the night the parody was on. After that, the network executives came back and said, "Okay forget it. You got everything you want. Come on over to ABC." It was a wonderful push for his career.

The Professor was influential in another way, as the inspiration for the Two Thousand Year Old Man, a celebrated series of interviews between a deadpan Reporter and a Mel Brooks character who was a different kind of expert, a character who'd been around so long he knew all of recorded history.

The Two Thousand Year Old Man was actually born on Max Liebman's couch. Carl turned to Mel one day and asked, "Did you know Jesus?"

"Oh boy," Mel said.

"You knew Jesus?"

"Thin boy. He used to come into the

store with twelve friends. Never bought anything. Just asked for a glass of water."

The tribute to the Professor that meant the most to me, however, was when I learned that one of the people who really identified with him was the greatest professor in the world.

We were at rehearsal for an installment of *Caesar's Hour* on a Friday, just a day before the show, and I was on the floor directing the scenery and the performers when my secretary came to me and said, "Dr. Einstein wants to talk to you." I said, "Okay fellas, very funny," looking at the writers and thinking that they'd put her up to it. But she said, "No, really. Albert Einstein is trying to get in touch with you." I still couldn't get it through my head. It was like getting a call from Copernicus. Even in the farthest reaches of my mind, I didn't believe that he would even know that I existed.

I went to my office and spoke with Helen Dukas, who took care of Dr. Einstein at the time. She told me that he would like to make an appointment to talk to me in his home in Princeton. I started to stammer. "He wants to talk to me? About what? What do I know that he doesn't know?"

I was stunned. I told my secretary, "Get me all the books about Einstein and physics you can find. I want to bone up on the theory of relativity over the weekend." But before we could schedule an appointment, he passed away in 1955. It was a great disappointment for me.

People who make great, great discoveries are always remembered, in art as well as science. We are always going to learn more and we are going to build on those discoveries. If you're still accepted years and years later that means you've accomplished something important. Einstein's $e=mc^2$ will always be remembered.

Years later, while lecturing at Columbia University, I was walking down a hall when a slim man approached me. "Pardon me," he said, "you're Sid Caesar, aren't you?"

"Yes I am."

"Let me introduce myself," the man said. "I'm Robert Oppenheimer. You know, Albert liked your work very much. He had mastered the physical equation, but he always wanted to talk to you about the human equation." I thanked Dr. Oppenheimer for sharing that with me.

Maybe the Professor was an authority on something after all.

Chapter 11

THE GERMAN GENERAL AND THE MUSIC OF DOUBLE-TALK

Without music, I don't think I would have been as creative — or as successful — as I was. Because comedy is timing, which includes rhythm, my skills as a musician inevitably gave me a tempo that was integral to my performing. But what the music also made me understand is that I could use melody in comedy. Melody is what brings everything together. The best thing you can do when you get a sketch is immediately memorize it, make the words second nature as soon as you can. Because once that happens you can play around with it the way a musician looks for nuances or variations on a theme.

There is a distinct rhythm to comedy, which is why when you are doing a live show you can't stop thirty or forty times. You can't break the rhythm. That's what ties the pieces, the sketches, and the players together.

372

Plus the rhythms are distinctly different from sketch to sketch. If you're going to do a sketch about a Spanish matador, then the tempo is very vibrant, like Bizet's *Carmen* or Ravel's *Bolero*, because it's all gesture. But if you're doing a husband in a domestic sketch, the rhythms are more normal. The diamond ring sketch, you'll remember, had a dramatic undertone to it. It's a serious matter, but it's also very funny. The audience knows I'm sitting with the ring in my pocket, my wife is running all over the apartment panicking because she thinks she lost it, and I'm getting more and more nervous over the chaos and the pain I'm causing her. The rhythm here is both anxious and funny.

The more time I spent in television, the more I thought about rhythm in terms of the overall show, not just individual sketches. Sometimes the tempos in one sketch would be too powerful for one beside it. They just didn't flow. When that happened, the running order of sketches had to go out the window.

Celebrating or parodying music and musical pieces also created the core of many of our sketches.

I did a satire of a pianist playing Grieg's *Piano Concerto in A Minor*. Without a piano. All I had was a bench. I came out in a white tie and tails, I bowed very deeply to the audience. I then flipped my tails and sat down on that bench and played the concerto with some extra hand flourishes here and there to make it funny.

The giant screen over the stage in the Century Theater was a big help for this sketch. It allowed us to do the pantomime for real, so the theatrical audience could see every move and nuance and react to the close-up shots the same way the television audience could.

At the end of the piece, I got up and took a bow. And people loved it. They thought I'd been playing the piano. There were actually arguments over it! Because I'd had musical training, I was able to get the simulation to the point where the audience thought it was real. They saw it in their mind's eye and the response was amazing. Once the show was over, wouldn't you know people told me they never knew I could play the piano so well. I said, "What are you talking about? There was no piano onstage!" Earl Wild, one of the greatest interpreters of Gershwin, was playing the piano backstage. No one wanted to believe it. Earl, in his late eighties, is still performing concerts and recording albums.

We also took on operas and made them comedic, which wasn't easy. So many people are intimidated or turned off by opera because they think it's so complex and highbrow. All it is is a story set to music. By parodying these classic tales, we demystified them. We actually introduced millions of people to opera and made it not only less threatening but inviting. By demystifying opera, I'll bet we introduced more people to that kind of music than all the PBS specials in history.

Earl Wild, who was then a staff pianist at ABC, also helped us with the operas. Earl auditioned for me and I knew he was gifted. We came up with our own version of *Pagliacci*, where we turned the crying clown whose wife has betrayed him for another man into someone called "Galipacci."

The challenge to performing operas was the arias. I didn't think I could memorize and learn the music in less than a week. Earl Wild solved the problem for us. He played a classical introduction to the tune of "Pop Goes the Weasel" and unlocked the operas for us. Setting the arias to the tunes of popular songs was the key to doing operas for us. It made it easier for everyone in the company to learn the music in the short time we had. It meant we didn't have to learn new melodies each week. It was also funny. I was so happy, I kissed him right on the forehead.

We used all kinds of tunes in "Galipacci," from "Santa Claus Is Coming to Town" for the opening to "Take Me Out to the Ball Game." Any Italian we needed was done in double-talk. The denouement, the moment of truth, comes with Howie saying, "Atsa show business." And as my love lay dying in my arms, we all sang to the great classical tune "The Yellow Rose of Texas."

Nanette had a wonderful operatic voice, and one of Carl's life dreams had been to become an opera singer. The only thing that stood in his way was that he was pretty much tone-deaf. There was only one note that Carl needed to hit here and he said, "I'll have a trumpet player give me that note." "Forget the trumpet," I said, "the whole orchestra is going to give you the note." And they did, but right before Carl was ready to hit it, one of the chorus girls standing next to him sneezed, and that's the note he took. The whole orchestra meant nothing.

The opera pieces always involved a lot of scenery, performers, and artists all working together. Our version of *The Count of Monte Cristo*, the classic Dumas story that's been made into a movie more than a dozen times, was especially elaborate. We used six easily recognizable tunes and turned it into an Italian opera, "The Count of Monte Clifto" by Giuseppi Vespucci — the favorite opera of Alfonso the First, the famous tone-deaf king.

I play the future count. We opened to the tune of "The Good Ship Lollipop" and then I court the lovely Rosella to the tune of "Tomatoes Are Cheaper, Potatoes Are Cheaper, Let's Fall in Love," all in Italian double-talk. Once I succeed in convincing her that "two can a live as cheap as one," I announce the wedding to the court: "No presents, just bring cash."

Carl plays the Fernand Mondego character who betrays me and has me jailed. I warn Rosa in song, also in Italian double-talk: "Ah Rosa, no fool arounda with the fellas when I'm in a cell'a, I'll breaka your nose-a." Howie Morris plays the Abee Faria character, the wise old man who teaches me art, history, and how to fence in prison. Our name for him was Mickey Mouse. I put my arm around Howie and we sang the M-I-C-K-E-Y song and gave the mouseketeer salute a few times during the sketch, which the audience absolutely went crazy over. Even Walt Disney wasn't safe from us. Then Howie swung the ball chained to his ankle into the wall to the tune of "Ballin' the Jack" and created an instant escape route, all in classical style.

"The third act is a television first," our narrator, Ben Grauer, tells the audience, "because no one has ever sat through the third act." "Somebody's gotta die," I say with vengeance in my heart. I turned to Howie: "I see ya in the finale." "Oh sure, I'll be there," he replies. All this to the tune of "Makin' Whoopee."

The finale is a sword fight between Carl and me. We are warming up with our swords. When he calls "en garde!" I take out a gun and shoot him. Indiana Jones stole that move from us years later. Carl keeps singing from the floor, so I keep shooting him. It was all done to the tune of "Hooray for Hollywood."

Because I'd played jazz, I enjoyed parodying it as much as classical music. We started with a character named Kool Seas, a jazz musician with a six-inch-thick buzz cut and Coke bottle glasses. I mean his reading glasses were two-foot long tubes. The character initially appeared as a pure musical sketch, "Flyin' Away in F." I got to play both the saxophone and the clarinet. With Larry Gelbart's brilliant ear for dialogue, we were able to capture Kool Seas' unique voice.

The next time we did Kool Seas, it was as an interview sketch. With Carl as Aristotle Cookie, the host of "Ominous," asking the questions, it was pure comedy:

Aristotle: We're here to talk about contemporary modern jazz with Mr. Kool Seas.
Kool: I'm happy to be here. Because if I wasn't here, I could be someplace else, where I'd be in danger.
Aristotle: Is it true that jazz originated before World War I?
Kool: There was a war?
Aristotle: Yes.
Kool: How did we come out?
Aristotle: We won.
Kool: Solid.
Aristotle: Can we continue with our discussion?
Kool: Yes, sir, I'd be most emaciated to.
Aristotle: When did jazz begin?
Kool: A million years ago. The world was full of volcanoes and the world was too hot not to cool down. Only birds could live. It was called Birdland.
Aristotle: How many men are in your band?

Kool: Fifteen men and a gorilla.
Aristotle: Why do you need the gorilla?
Kool: He's the only one who can drive the bus.
Aristotle: Do you see any good in rock and roll?
Kool: Only if we could divert the energy for peaceful purposes.

Kool Seas became Progress Hornsby after we got a letter from a teacher in Baltimore. All of her students were sight impaired and wore thick glasses. She thought the character was making fun of the students. As soon as I got the letter, I wrote an apology back and then told the writers, "Fellas, we have to change the character. We're not out to hurt anyone, especially children." I took off the glasses, smoothed out the hair, and put on a ruffled shirt with lace cuffs. That was how the too-hip Progress Hornsby was born. It was Carl again, as Ted Burrows (a take-off on Edward R. Murrow), who interviewed Progress.

Ted: Good evening. I am Ted Burrows and this is "People to People." Tonight we are going to Chicago to talk to one of the leading exponents in the modern school of jazz, Mr. Progress Hornsby. Mr. Hornsby lives in this modest apartment in Chicago. Good evening, Mr. Hornsby.

Progress: And hello to whoever is saying hello to me.

Ted: It's nice of you to have us, Mr. Hornsby. Tell us, how do you like being in Chicago?

Progress: It's the world's most man. Haven't you heard? They put out the fire. It's cool here.

Ted: When were you born?

Progress: I would be most hermetically sealed to tell you, sir. I was born in 1927. February the 68th.

Ted: Did you say February the 68th?

Progress: Yes sah, that was a leap year. And we really leaped that year! We segued from February to October, thereby avoiding the hot weather and making the whole year cool. You know what I mean?

Ted: You have a most unusual hairstyle.

Progress: Yes, it does have a touch of the Ming Dynasty, doesn't it?

Ted: Progress, how do you get your barber to cut your hair?

Progress: I insult him. And this is his revenge. But I love it.

Ted: How often do you have your hair cut?

Progress: I have my hair cut only once a year.

Ted: Only once a year?

Progress: So I can save it. I'm wearing it now, sir. This suit is me. You've heard of mohair? This is me-hair.

Ted: Can we get on with our discussion of jazz?

Progress: I would be most hydraulically lifted to, sir.

Ted: Isn't it true that jazz originated in New Orleans before World War I?

Progress: There was a war?

Ted: Yes.

Progress: How did we come out?

Ted: We won.

Progress: Solid.

Ted: Progress, I know that you have been playing for a good many years. Have you ever played Europe?

Progress: Who published it?

Ted: No, I mean Europe the continent across the ocean. Progress, I know that you've played with all the old time jazz greats. Who is the most outstanding of them all?

Progress: Well, without a doubt, man. It's Peter "Fats" Fidelio.

Ted: The great trumpet man who was the first man to hit a C above high C.

Progress: That's the legend, man. But the truth is that it was here in the apartment ten years ago that Fats blew a high M.

Ted: An M? I thought the scale stopped at G.

Progress: Not for the brave, sir. You see, Fats was courageous. He hit an M then went for a high R above S.

Ted: What happened to him?

Progress: Fats Fidelio has become the first space station. He blew himself out of this world. He is now circling the earth in a fine tempo. Look, there he goes now.

Ted: I understand you've completed a new album.

Progress: Yes, it's on the Condemned Label.

Ted: I understand it's on a special sort of hi-fi.

Progress: Oh, man, this is the highest they've ever fied. If they fi any higher than this, they're gonna foo! And if they foo, I want to be there when they do, man!

Ted: It's too bad we can't have a sample of your music.

Progress: Oh, I always have a band in my apartment. What's a musician without a band?

Ted: Tell me, Progress, what do you call your band?

Progress: We call ourselves the Guy Lombardo Orchestra. We get a lot of work that way. Otherwise we'd starve instantly.

Ted: Progress, can we meet the members of your band?

Progress: Wishing will make it so. On the first trumpet we have the late Fats Fidelio, on the 88s we have Johnson 66, on the bongos we have the incredible Johnny Shrinko, and on the siren we have Pop Screaming Yo-Yo. And we have the inevitable Cinco Barrata on radar.

Ted: You have radar in the band?

Progress: Oh, *très nécessaire,* sir. Whenever we play, we must be warned in case we approach the melody.

Ted: What are you going to play for us this evening?

Progress: Our latest recording, a song that has not been heard anywhere: "The National Anthem of the Moon."

It was my love of jazz that also led to the Haircuts, our takeoff on '50s rock and roll groups. One time when I went down to Birdland in Manhattan to hear George Shearing, the strangest relief band came out between sets. They were so high they didn't know where the hell they were. They may have all started at the same time, but I don't think they ever played in the same key, or even the same song.

After that a singing trio came out. All three guys were dressed in the same outfit: zoot suits with the big lapel handkerchiefs hanging out. And their hair hung right above their eyebrows. They may have had a different name, but they became the Haircuts to me.

Those guys sang very simple songs, which is why we wrote the Haircut lyric, "You are so rare to me, oh very rare to me. So if I'm rare to you, won't you be rare." That was it, and it was actually longer than the song the guys in the relief band sang. As soon as we saw it, we worked on the characters. We rehearsed the thing for a week and then the Haircuts made their national debut. On the other side of the record, the flip side, we created "Going Crazy." We said "You Are So Rare to Me" was selling more than "Going Crazy," so we said "we're only going to sell half a record." We loved doing the group because coming up with a fifth sketch every week was very difficult.

On *Caesar's Hour*, I got to play with Benny Goodman, which was one of the highlights of my musical and professional career. To reunite with Benny in this way was a great joy.

I've always considered double-talk to be

a form of music as well, with each language having its own rhythm. One day in the Writers' Room, Carl started speaking in Italian double-talk, and I realized that this could become a sketch. Carl sold me a package of cigarettes in Italian as a tryout, and it worked beautifully. So was born the foreign movie sketch. We now had another area of comedy we could develop and explore.

In the ongoing search for material, the writers and I would leave the theater every Friday afternoon at 4:00 p.m. to see foreign films at the Museum of Modern Art on 53rd Street. We had finished the run-through with the technical guys, the musical choruses are being rehearsed, and it was a good time for us to take a break. The museum would have a run of films starring Clark Gable, Mae West, Cary Grant, or great European actors like Emil Jannings and Harry Bauer. Seeing all those films put us right in the mood. The writers and I also made a habit of coordinating the choice of dining with whatever foreign movie we were working on.

We did movies in Italian, French, German, and Japanese double-talk. We never wrote double-talk out word for word, we just laid out the goals, the comic direction.

Most of our actions were similar to the movies we were parodying. That, coupled with mannerisms and gestures, as well as a few English words thrown in, gave the audience a clear idea of what was going on. You had to make yourself understood.

The foreign movies took on a life of their own and developed a very strong following. Our set designer, Freddy Fox, was in Philadelphia one Saturday night at a theater, working on a show he had designed the scenery for. There was a bar right next door to the theater. During the intermission, everyone went next door for a drink. The bartender, who was Italian, had *Your Show of Shows* on, and we'd already announced that we were doing a parody of the Italian movie *La Bicicletta* (*The Bicycle Thief*).

The bartender yelled out, "Okay, everybody order up because there's gonna be an Italian movie on and there will be no service until it's over." Freddy sat there and watched in awe as the bartender then sat down at the bar as the Italian movie parody unfolded and proceeded to translate what I was saying on the air in my Italian double-talk to the customers at the bar. Freddy looked around. People were actually listening intently to the bartender interpreting the movie.

In our parody, I said, "I want to introduce you to my wife," and Imogene came out dressed like Anna Magnani, with a big wig and a fancy little peasant dress and again acted like she was the sexiest woman in the world. She fell right into the role. The audience rocked and rolled.

I had just seen my first Japanese movie, *Gate of Hell*, which won the best foreign language Oscar in 1954 and was the first Japanese film widely released in the United States. Japanese, to me, sounds a lot like German. We were inspired to marry this Japanese movie with the legends about King Arthur and his court. Japanese movies like that were only playing in major cities like New York and San Francisco, but the larger audience got the story, and it was funny.

"Take-a-Kuki Productions Presents *Ubetu*" took its name from *Ugetsu* by director Kenji Mizoguchi, Kurosawa's predecessor. I played Shtaka Yamagura, a samurai warrior. "This is a legend of ancient Japan," the narration began, "set in the fourteenth century when powerful warlords ruled the country with the help of samurai warriors." Samurai warriors who said things like "Sun Yat Sen, at's some gong" and "You bow like a cow."

The emperor, Mashashima, played by Howie, intends to reward his warriors with anything they wish. I have my eye on his daughter, Latatoto, "a tender maiden of high birth," played by Nanette. So does my rival, Goshinoto, played by Carl, naturally.

As the brave warriors return from battle, they hastily sheathe their swords. Legend has it if a warrior draws his sword in the palace, he brings dishonor on himself and his family. Goaded by Goshinoto, ("Whatsa matta wit me? Whatsa matta wit you!") Shtaka commits the one unforgivable sin — he removes his sword from its scabbard. Now he's lost his honor, his titles, and his maiden. Naturally, he vows to recapture them.

I realize that I have been tricked into unsheathing my sword, and I challenge Carl to a duel. Carl and I dance around each other with our swords drawn. "You scared," I ask in a Japanese accent. "I scared," he replies.

When my sword gets stuck in a tree stump and I cannot remove it, Carl smiles thinking he can now kill me. I uproot the entire stump with my sword still in it and hit Carl on the head. "At'sa concussion!" Carl exclaims as he falls to the ground in defeat. Shtaka reclaims his honor and wins the hand of the lovely Latatoto.

When our samurai were dueling, it sounded like someone was yelling "Whazzup!" My brothers Dave and Abe were extras in the sketch, playing giant samurai warriors. We interspersed Yiddish words like shmo, which sounded Japanese, into the dialogue. We used a lot of Yiddish words for character names because they were just funny: Baron Kasha, Gantza Metzia (which means "big deal"), which also sounds Japanese if you say it right. I am pretty sure I'm responsible for introducing the word "chutzpah" into the American vernacular. I remember looking for the right word in a sketch and blurting out, "That guy has an awful lot of chutzpah!"

One of our satires in German was a movie about the heroic fliers of what we called the Richtenflichten Flying Circus led by the great Ricky Richtofen. "Der Flying Ace," our German World War I movie, took place in 1915 in "zum place on der vestern front." The credits mentioned writer Field Marshall von Kaltvasser, director General von Klipstein, and associate producer General von Krupdingle. If the double-talk Yiddish sounded funny, it went in.

"In des hohres 1915 die German Armeen sind raus gemoved, die vurld zu conqueren. Ein wichitiger important teil of diewser Armeen var die Airforce oder die Lufftwaffe. Die var aufgemacht up of lunge manner, oder die creamsahne des German Beuolherungeren populace. . . . Und dot's dot."

Howie was Lieutenant von Schplitz, who boasted "un geplots tzvi Englishe planar." As the planes sputter, there are raspberry sound effects in the background. Carl is the old-fashioned Lieutenant von Schissel. "Hab a little reschpect for da var. Du bist nischt ein pilot, du bist a ninety-day vunder."

Howie mourns my apparent death. "Richtofen — Ricky — Ricky aut geplattzed. Ricky got exploded. Ein schveet fella."

I walk in — miraculously alive. "Who gepacked the parachute? Aut fallen twelve thousand feet on my helmet."

I unveil a secret weapon, which I can't pro-nounce, zeppelin, dirigible, whatever. Let's call it a blimp. "We're bombing London," I announce. "Ver is London?" is the reply. Once on the blimp (which has a neon sign saying "Drink Kaiser's beer"), we announce "bombs avec" and away they went.

One of our most famous satires, "The

German General" sketch, was largely a combination of two movies, one American and one German.

The American film was *Blind Husbands*, which starred the great actor Erich von Stroheim as a German officer on a mountain climbing vacation in Austria. Only one day he didn't climb. While his partner climbed the mountain, he seduced his partner's wife. He also wore a uniform with fifteen Iron Crosses and epaulets on the shoulders. He used two military brushes to shine his bald head. In *Grand Illusion*, another film, von Stroheim played an officer so aristocratic someone else blew into his gloves before he put them on.

The other main film was *The Last Laugh*, which starred Emil Jannings as the very proud doorman at a very fancy Berlin hotel who was especially enamored of his ornate uniform. In those days, Germans were all about uniforms; doormen had nicer uniforms than generals did — more braid, better looking caps. The Jannings character had no power or prominence outside the hotel. His biggest boast was that he could handle any piece of luggage known to man. His life was his job. He even wore the uniform home.

One night during a rainstorm, a big

Duesenberg drives up with a huge trunk on top. Because of the rain, the trunk is too heavy to hold. The doorman drops it and there is a dent. The manager takes him to the office and yells at him. "You realize what has happened?" The doorman apologizes profusely to the trunk's owner and the manager but to no avail. He pleads for his job. The manager takes him off the door and makes him the men's room attendant. Talk about dejected. The man was so depressed he would steal the doorman's uniform and wear it home every night so no one would know of his demotion. In his mind, he had gone from the prestigious top job to the undignified bottom.

This was a film with two endings, and in Europe they showed both of them. The first ending has him broken, tending to people as the men's room attendant, getting penny tips. In the alternate ending, a rich man befriends him, rescues him from the men's room, and gives him a job. He now checks into the hotel as a guest, calls the manager over and says, "The suite is not up to my standards."

In the sketch, I played a very arrogant German general. Howie played my sycophantic and barely competent manservant, who helps dress me with my boots, coat, buttons, epaulets, and medals. He polishes my buttons, spitting on each one. In his zeal he sprays me in the eye. "Du ast geschprizzed on de General?" I complain, astonished.

Howie breathes heavily on my monocle. ("Das monocle ist geschmutzik!") He breathes a little too hard, until it's "schlippery from schaliva!" He takes off my robe and scarf, puts a tunic on me, buttons it, and polishes the buttons. Then he clips my collar, but too tightly: "Du hasta klipt der shkin!"

He flicks the strands of epaulets ("Epaulets flicken!"), attaches the braids ("Ba-raid rest!"). He blows into both gloves and slips one on each hand. As he polishes my medals (including the Blue Cross, the Medal of Honor, and the one for the fifty-yard dash), I say, "Du hasta jinglen der medalen? Du bist a medal jingler?"

Howie then hides behind the mirror. When I stand before the mirror to look at myself, asking, "Mirror mirror on the wall, who's the schlickest one of all?" in a high voice he responds, "You are, General."

Howie moves on to the "perfume spritzen" and puts on my cap backward. "Du machen da fool here?" I yell. We right the cap. Now the general is "der schlickest one of all" and ready for work. The payoff is that I walk out of the dressing room in full ceremonial dress into another room where everyone is in evening clothes. I then go outside through the revolving door where an elegantly dressed couple follows. We exchange pleasantries, and then I take off one of my braids, which is a whistle. I blow the whistle and hail a cab for them. The general is a doorman!

Because foreign movies were only shown in the big cities, we were ahead of the curve in our creativity. But we never played down to the audience. In 1955 Charles Berlitz of the Berlitz School of Languages presented me with an award on the air. "For all the fun in foreign languages that you've shown us through the years," he said, "We are presenting you with an Award of Merit." It's true, we probably did as much as anyone to promote interest in other languages. But as I told the audience that night, when we did foreign films I had more fun than anyone else. Which I did.

Chapter 12

"FROM HERE TO OBSCURITY," "AGGRAVATION BOULEVARD," AND OTHER MOVIE SATIRES

After fifty years, movie satires are still a staple of television. I would have a lot of fun as Batman, Spider-Man, James Bond, or Indiana Jones. From the inception, we were constantly on the lookout for something, anything we could use. So if a great movie came out, we would all go and see it and figure out if we could do a parody.

These kinds of sketches were high on my list because I always loved movies, whether they were great or not. Our wide-ranging taste meant that nothing was safe. One week I was Zorro, making Xs instead of Zs on my victims. Another week I was Samson ("Excuse me, there's a crazy woman after me with a pair of scissors"). In *The King and I*, dressed up as a barefoot

Yul Brynner stepping on a lit cigarette, I was yelling, "How many times I gotta tell ya, no smokin' in the palace!" In a takeoff on prison movies, I played an escaped convict who climbs to the top of the wall. The warden shines the spotlight on me, and in my best Jolson, I break into a chorus of "One bright and shining light . . . that taught me wrong from right . . ."

Nothing was too obscure for us. We even did a sketch parodying bullfighting movies. I played the champion matador, Flamingo, who had unaccountably left the ring. Carl played the up-and-coming star who mercilessly taunts me: "You always fight in small towns — Madrid . . . Levittown! Flamingo, you are a coward, you are a sissy, and you only fight lady bulls!"

"I have gone into a new business," I tell him. "Children's ready-to-wear. Why I quit is only between me and the bulls, and I don't want to tell you about it."

Finally Carl's taunts get me back into the ring. Immy plays my girlfriend who sobs, "I can't watch the fight."

"You must watch the fight," I insist. "Here is a ticket." She takes my arm. After looking lovingly into each other's eyes, I say, "That will be $1.85. It's a mezzanine, you know. The bulls are not mad at us, they are out to make a living, like us."

The challenge in all our movie parodies was to find the delicate balance between capturing the flavor of the movie and at the same time creating a new piece. The satire had to work for the part of the audience that had already seen the movie and the other part that hadn't. If you hear the underlying piece in your head, then you can do the parody.

Satires could be complicated in other ways. Jack Benny got in trouble for doing an exact copy of the movie *Gaslight* on radio. The Supreme Court had ruled you couldn't parody word for word or scene for scene, so we didn't. We would never parody a movie that had social merit, like *The Life of Emile Zola*, or a movie that wasn't a hit. And we would never do a satire of a bad movie because bad is bad. If you started out with a bad movie, the parody would never get funnier than what you were starting out with. The better a movie was, the more material we were able to find. We also learned that if we parodied a movie there was a good chance that it would become a hit because of all the attention that it got.

"On the Docks," our parody of *On the Waterfront*, almost didn't get on the air at all. *On the Waterfront* had just opened on Broadway. It was a low-budget picture even for those days, made for about $300,000. It was only doing a little business, but when we saw it we knew it was ripe for a satire.

Right before the show, I got a phone call from the producer, Sam Spiegel. Spiegel had also produced *The African Queen*. He was ashamed of his Jewish background and liked to call himself S. P. Eagle. He had heard about the parody and he blustered over the phone, "If you make fun of my movie on your show, I'll sue the hell out of you."

Naturally, we called our lawyers. They didn't tell us we couldn't do the sketch but didn't assure us that we wouldn't have a lawsuit. We had already built the sets and created the costumes, and because we figured it would cost us the same amount of money to cancel the sketch as it would to litigate, we decided to go ahead and do it. The sketch worked out very well. "On the Docks" had a texture to it that was true to the movie, that captured Elia Kazan's tone. I played the Marlon Brando part of the young dockworker, using my patented technique of "Method mumbling." I was able to capture his movements with a quick flick of my hips.

Carl played the Rod Steiger role of my brother Charlie. When Carl asks me if I'm gonna squeal, I assure him that I'll never talk to anyone. "You told me never to talk to anyone, and I didn't. I never even talked to Mom and Pop, but I wished I did. They seemed like such nice people." We didn't cast anyone in Karl Malden's priest role; we didn't want to make fun of religion in any way. Also, not using every character protected us from potential copyright violation.

Nanette played the Eva Marie Saint role, the girl from the neighborhood. Howie played her father, a dockworker killed by my racketeer brother. When I go to visit Nanette, I keep knocking on her door and she won't let me in. Finally, I break through the wall with my bare hands. We begin to kiss passionately though Nanette protests by hitting me on the head repeatedly with a hammer, first violently, then more softly, and finally lovingly stroking my hair with the hammer.

During our love scene on the roof where I raised pigeons, I keep asking her, "You sure you're not a cop? I never kissed a cop before. I don't want to get no reputation as a cop kisser." Getting more personal, I tell her about how poor I was growing up.

Sid: You know how poor I was when I was a kid? I'm gonna be truthful witcha. I never tasted a tangerine. I never tasted a tangerine to this day. Never had fruit in the house. No fruit in the house!
Nanette: You poor guy. You never had anybody to show you any kindness or any kind of affection at all, did you?
Sid: It's a miracle I didn't end up with scurvy!

The *New York Times* picked up that line in its review.

When Carl points the gun at me at the climax, there is briefly no dialogue. We waited for the audience. Unlike the famous "I could'a been a contenda" scene between Steiger and Brando, Carl starts shooting at me and keeps missing. "You're a good person, you have a good soul, but you know why you can't hit me, because you're cockeyed," I tell him. There was some wonderful business in that sketch. If you're not interrupted, you can build a rhythm. And because it was live, we were in charge of our own timing and delivery.

The week after the satire aired, you couldn't get near the movie theater. The

401

lines were around the block. I got another phone call.

"Mr. Caesar, this is Mr. S. P. Eagle."

"Yes, Mr. Eagle," I said, expecting the worst.

"Mr. Caesar I have another script called *The Bridge on the River Kwai*. I could send it over to you. Or I can send you a copy of the first print. I could also have Alec Guinness and William Holden come over and perform scenes for you." Not one word about the lawsuit. That's what you call a switch. Four days ago he was going to sue me, and now he wants to give me a script. Ats'a show business!

That was the power of satire and the impact we had on America at the time. People saw the satires, which were funny in and of themselves, and then they wanted to see the originals.

Marlon Brando also called after "On the Docks" aired. When I picked up the phone, I expected him to come on yelling. He just said "Now, that was funny," and then he hung up.

One of the first satires of an American movie we did was George Stevens's *A Place in the Sun*, with Elizabeth Taylor, Montgomery Clift, and Shelly Winters. Ours was called "A Place in the Bottom of the

Lake" and focused on the scene where Clift's character, played by me, thinks about killing his old girlfriend, played by Immy, in the middle of Maloon Lake. But first, Carl Reiner, who played the voice of my interior monologue, sets the scene.

"Fifty years ago the movies had no sound at all. Nowadays, the sound track of a movie brings you not only the voices of the actors, but another very important effect . . . Music! And as if that isn't enough a lot of movies now bring us . . . the voice of the actor's conscience. Tonight we're going to bring you a typical Hollywood movie, complete with music, drama, and a voice that will tell you just what the leading man is thinking."

After sneaking a knife, a gun, a dingle-dangle, a chain, and an anchor onto the boat, I begin to wrestle with both my conscience and a very dim-witted yet love-struck Immy.

Coca: When are we going to get married, Montgomery? Let's get married today. Why can't we get married today, Montgomery? You'll see, Montgomery, it's going to be real nice. We'll have a real nice apartment with real nice furniture and real nice carpets and real nice curtains at the window and a real nice kitchen and everything will be real nice! Maybe we won't have much money. Maybe we'll be poor and we'll have to struggle, but it'll be nice. Montgomery . . . Whatta you thinking?

Carl: (on mike) This girl is an idiot. How did I ever get mixed up with her?

Sid: Nothing.

Coca: Oh Montgomery, when we're married, I'll wait on you hand and foot. I'll be a slave to you!

Sid: Gee Mildred, you won't have to do that.

Carl: (on mike) I can't kill her. She loves me.

Coca: I love you, Montgomery.

Carl: (on mike) You see?

Coca: I'll take such good care of you! I'll see that you wear your rubbers when it rains, and I'll see that you go to sleep early every night. I'll bring your lunch pail to work every day and I'll phone you every hour to make sure you're all right, and I'll call for you after work every day and I'll never let you out of my sight . . .

Carl: (on mike) I've got to kill this girl! This girl has got to go!

Sid: Look at the pretty water lilies, Mildred.

(Music) (She looks)

Carl: (on mike) Now's your chance! Take out the gun! Take out the cartridges! Load the gun! Come on! Whattaya doing? You put the bullets in the wrong way! Hurry up! Not the rope you fool! The gun! That's the knife! Whattaya doing? Come on, butterfingers!

Sid: I only got two hands!

Coca: What did you say, Montgomery?

Sid: (Hiding the gun) I said I'm making big plans, and they include you! (Music)

Coca: Gee, just think, Montgomery, by this time tomorrow we'll be married!

Sid: I'm thinking, I'm thinking!

Westerns were also ripe for satire, and we did takeoffs on several. One of my favorites was *Shane*, which we called "Strange." My first name is Very, but I tell people they can call me Strange. I show up in town and start to drink from a barrel of water with a ladle. I take twenty or thirty swallows. I tip the barrel to drink even more. When I swagger away, you can hear the water sloshing around in my stomach. Immy, playing the young Brandon de Wilde character, says, "You seem mighty thirsty. Have a long, dry ride?" "No," I answer. "I had a herring for breakfast."

We also did a parody of John Ford's

Stagecoach called "No West for the Wicked," which we called "a story of valor and courage on Saddle Soap Theater." Carl played Randolph Snide, Howie was the Gabby Hayes character, and I was Johnny Jingo, the John Wayne character. Ominous music follows each mention of my name. I have drawn my last gun and killed my last man. I'm trying to leave town, so that people won't know that I'm the greatest, but the old ways die hard.

"There's three women on that stage," someone tells me, "and one of them is having a baby."

"I ain't looking for trouble, but if that baby wants it, I'll give it to him."

High Noon was a different kind of story. It was a very simple, beautiful black-and-white picture that builds up to a wonderful climax. It was a big hit, so there was definitely some meat there to play with.

I played the Gary Cooper role of the sheriff who has to defend his town against gunslingers all by himself because no one will help him. "How can you stay here and wait for a man to come and kill you," I am asked. "Cause I'm stupid," is my sober reply. I mumbled to myself the way Gary Cooper would. The whole idea was to take an actor's style and movements and exaggerate them.

Each time one of the deputies came in and told me they couldn't help, they were supposed to apologize and then pin their badge back on me. Things, however, didn't go exactly as planned.

The costumer had prepared a big sponge pad, which was supposed to go under my shirt. As I rushed out of the dressing room, I saw the sponge out of the corner of my eye. But they were playing the opening music for the sketch and there was no time to go back.

The deputies weren't real actors; they were kids from the chorus. When each of the deputies came in to give the badge back, I kept saying "No, no, no, no, no," but they thought I was just ad-libbing in the scene. The first deputy said, "I'd love to help you, Sheriff, but my wife is pregnant and she wants me to be home with her." And wham — the badge was pinned into my skin. Each badge had a pin that was an inch and a half long. I grimaced in pain. The next guy came up and said, "Sheriff, my wife wants to go to a dance tonight, and I'm sorry." Wham! Another badge pinned into my skin. And I kept putting my hands up, going "No, no, no, no, no." The third guy came in and I threw my arms up and said, "Go ahead." You can't fight destiny. After the show, the writers came backstage and said, "Wow, Sid, we knew you could do great pain takes, but those were really good." "Fellas," I said, "they were for real." I opened my shirt and said, "Look at the holes. I need a tetanus shot." I really did. The doctor was already on his way.

Over the course of the years, we parodied *The Rifleman, Have Gun, Will Travel, Gunsmoke, Bat Masterson* (renamed "Hat Basterson"), and *Wagon Train.* We may not have been the fastest guns in the West, but we were darn near the funniest, I reckon.

Speaking of tetanus shots, doctors weren't safe from us either. In our parody of Ben Casey–type shows, "Emergency," I played a devoted and very straitlaced surgeon. "He's using old-fashioned pills when the patient should be treated . . . psychiligically," I tell the chief of the hospital. "We are more than doctors, we are bulwarks of science. Somewhere in the body there is a place for the brain."

I recite the Hippocratic oath ad nauseam, adding, "I assure you that I am hip to my Hippocratic oath and all that jazz." I believe that was the first time that phrase, which Bob Fosse later made very famous as a musical, was introduced into the American vernacular. Immy played a patient with "a clear case of psychonomic amnesia." I am trying to restore her memory, and in the sketch she is submerged in a tank of water, where she starts to act like a seal.

In the sketch, a young woman, the head doctor's daughter, who is interested in me romantically, invites me to lunch at the club. "I cannot go with you," I say, "I just had some meatballs." She tries to leave in a huff. She had accidentally slammed the door so hard on her way in, it got stuck. It wouldn't open. She was yelling, and the audience was laughing.

"Why don't you go with her?" Carl asks.

"I don't think she knows which way she's going," I ad-libbed, which got an even bigger laugh. "By the way, the door don't open," I whispered not so silently to the crew. You never heard such loud trampling of feet on the other side of the door, as the stagehands rushed to get the door open.

One week, we did a parody of Kirk Douglas's *The Bad and the Beautiful*. We had every woman in the sketch with the same Veronica Lake peek-a-boo hairdo. I played a producer and Carl played an actor who was having an affair with one of my girls. I find out about the affair and I punch Carl. He literally flies around the room, going from table to lamp to table, breaking every piece of crockery in sight. He continued to fly into the next room and then into the living room, all based on one small punch.

Commercials weren't safe either. We even did a satire on a car commercial: "The 1957 Fiasco." That pretty much says it all.

We had fun with a lot of genre movies. Our spoof of spy pictures was called "Continental Express." I play a bumbling secret agent who can't hold on to secret papers (not unlike Maxwell Smart in Mel Brooks's later sitcom, *Get Smart*). "The ugly one gets the papers and the good-looking one is the rat," my chief tells me as I board the train to Istanbul on an under-cover assignment involving national security. Imogene, Carl, and Howie board my com-partment. Who is the ugly one and who is the good-looking one? I don't know who can be trusted.

When we go through a tunnel, the lights go out and there are sounds of fistfighting. (In the Writers' Room, we called these "light-ups" rather than blackouts.) When the lights come back on, my secret papers are gone. "All right. Who's the wise guy?" I ask. We go into another tunnel. The lights go off again, and there is even more commotion. When the lights come back up, my pants are gone. "Let's act like adult spies, please," I ask everyone.

In another spy sketch on a train, I sell some secret plans for 2 million zlotnies. Cash. What a deal. When I get off the train ecstatic and go to buy a newspaper, I throw a couple of zlotnies at the vendor. "Keep the change," I tell him. "You don't understand," he says. "The paper is 6 million zlotnies."

Hard-nosed newspaper movies were also a lot of fun to play. We did one called "Three Star Semi-Final" where I played two-fisted reporter Ace Johnson. Immy played Sob Sister Sally, a fellow reporter who's got the tough luck to be in love with a newshound like me. "You're not a man, you're a machine," she tells me. "You have printer's ink in your veins."

"Maybe that's why I get so nauseous," I reply.

We head for the Hi-Ho Club, on the trail of a gangster played by Carl and his "gorillas." There is an actual gorilla guarding the door. After a brief struggle with one of the gangsters, I end up with his gun. Holding everyone at gunpoint, I have the bad guys make change for me so I can use the pay phone to call the cops. It was such a kooky sketch.

Close in spirit to newspaper movies were the always popular gangster films. In "Bullets over Broadway" Nanette played Moxie, a cigarette girl in a club ("Cigars, cigarettes, bullets?") whose dream it is to someday be a singer in a cheap speakeasy. She breaks into her favorite song: "You can't put a price tag on love. It isn't smart, you'll get hurt. This is my heart, not a shirt."

I played the big boss, the Moose. "The Moose has ears like a hawk," one of my men says. "He can hear from blocks away." I walk into the club and say, "I was just in the barber shop a block away and I heard that." I fall in love with Nanette the moment I see her. When my old girlfriend complains, I smash a grapefruit in her face Jimmy Cagney style. Dave played a bartender in that scene.

Moxie tells me I am uncouth. "I ran a little short on couth," I tell her. I tell my men, "You guys go out and get all the couth you can get and bring it here. Take the big truck." Finding out that it's not that easy, I hire Professor Bernard Cyranno (Carl) to teach my men and me how to be couth. I recite what I've learned about history: "Napoleon — this guy was always ready. He always had his hand on his rod. Also, if you're a short gangster, stay away from tall Englishmen."

Bernard falls in love with Moxie. There is a showdown with a rival gang. As Moose lies dying, he takes his theater tickets — riddled with bullet holes — out of his breast pocket, and gives them to Bernard and Moxie. Thirty-eight years later Woody Allen called me. "I want to use the title 'Bullets over Broadway' for my new movie," he said, "and I want to make a deal with you."

"You just did," I told him. Because he came to me like a gentleman and asked for permission there was no way I was going to charge him. "Just make a great movie," I said. And he did.

"Prison Walls" was true to the George Raft films of the '30s and '40s. We spared no expense in the casting:

Cast
Prisoner 16078. . . . Clark Bigley
Prisoner 82093 . . . Bob Sanders
Prisoner 2345 . . . Sandy Roberts
Prisoner 14690 . . . . . Jim Clark
Prisoner 78965 . . . Robert James

413

And Starring
6789054321 75689025

Played by
3274

All numbers are fictitious and any resemblance to numbers living or dead is purely coincidental.

Howie, Carl, a few other actors, and I played convicts up the river at the state penitentiary:

Narrator: (Marching feet behind) The big rock! High gray walls enclosing a human volcano of turbulent emotions. Men paying for their crimes. Men without hope. Men without women. *Dangerous* men.
(Shot . . . Prison yard. Men milling around)
Guard: Halt! Awright! Rest period! (Shot . . . Carl, Howie, and three other prisoners saunter over to wall)
Carl: I hear they're letting Big Mike out of solitary today.
Howie: Yeah. Any minute now. He sure was in solitary a long time. Six months!
Carl: I'm surprised they're letting him out, after what he did.
Ray: That Big Mike — he sure is tough.

Howie: He was a big guy on the outside.

Carl: The stories he can tell! Boy . . . just before they put him in solitary he was telling us about this last job they pulled. They were robbing a bank in broad daylight when all of a sudden this crazy Indian walks in with a double-barreled shotgun.

Ray: What happened?

Carl: I don't know. That's when the fight started and they put him in solitary.

Howie: Hey! Here he comes! (They all look)

Carl: Gee, six months in solitary!

Howie: I wonder how he feels. (Music as Sid approaches, mean and tough, walks up to Carl)

Sid: So this crazy Indian walks in with a double-barreled shotgun . . . and we were left holding the bag. We were framed. Anybody got a butt? Gimme a butt!

Carl: Sure! I been saving it . . . but you can have it, Big Mike. (Gives it to him)

Howie: Here's a match I sneaked out of the kitchen.

Sid: Thanks, Stone Face. (Strikes match on Howie's face, lights up) Boys, while I was in solitary, I spent a lot of time thinking! I did a *lot* of thinking. I got a lot of thoughts. I thought about the walls . . . the bars . . . the guards with the guns. You know what I figured out?

Carl: What?

Sid: We're in prison.
Howie: He's right!

One of our favorite movies was Jules Dassin's caper movie *Rififi*, which he later remade into *Topkapi*. The film is famous for its twenty-five-minute silent sequence detailing an elaborate jewelry store robbery. In our version, Carl, Howie, and I played thieves trying to steal the "Bellini Cup," the only one of its kind in the world.

I play a wealthy man whose dream it is to steal the cup from the museum. I set out to assemble a team. I contact a ruffian from the street who leads me to the right crew. I go into the bathroom where Carl is literally taking a bath. "I'll give you £50 to help me steal the priceless cup. C'mon," I tell him, "we gotta go right now." "I'm with ya, gov." He got out of the tub immediately, already fully dressed in a suit. "How much is the cup worth?" he asks. "Never mind," I tell him.

Carl obviously needed to be dried off, but there could be no stopping the sketch — it was live. We had people off camera with towels and robes who patted him down as best they could — and he still had to do the rest of the sketch wet. To give them the time to dry as much as possible, we made Carl the last person in the next scene. Live necessitated a lot of planning.

Carl, Howie (whom I recruited as the dynamite man), and I wore sneakers with soles a foot thick, so we could be as stealthy as the thieves in the original film. We had to lean against things because the shoes were so hard to walk in. The sound engineers turned up the microphones so that every little sound could be heard. We pushed an inflatable raft through a hole in the wall into the museum and inflated it to catch the debris falling from our break-through. We began very carefully to drill through the wall. And then — here is the absurd part — we busted loudly through the wall in an explosion of bricks. We didn't dare talk; we had big signs. The Bellini Cup was on a pedestal with lights. I lifted the cup and triggered all of the alarms. I stuffed my hat in between the bell and the ringer, which stifled the entire intricate alarm system. At the end of the sketch we are in my opulent home, celebrating our good fortune. Each of us raised our glasses, toasted, drank, and tossed our glasses into the fireplace. I drank from the Bellini Cup and inadvertently tossed it into the fire-place, where it smashed. That was some ending.

We also did a takeoff on Broadway musicals (which was hardly surprising given the future Broadway playwrights in the Writers' Room) that was a combination of *42nd Street* and *A Star Is Born*. The sketch started out on a farm, with Nanette playing the young ingenue, Nancy Kidinthechorus, who keeps telling her grandmother, "I have to go to Broadway. I've got to sing, I've got to dance. I've got to show them what I can do." Her grandmother isn't impressed. "Ah my dear, it's not worth it. Stay on the farm, settle down, you'll be set for life. I was on Broadway," she says, and then the old woman starts doing acrobatic moves, tumbling and turning.

I played Maurice, the hyperactive Broadway producer who's opening a new show. "I'll sew the costumes for the elephants myself," I say. "After that, I'll paint the scenery. The show is running too long — take out the intermission!" He ran every aspect of the production.

Nancy auditions and gets a small part. On opening night, the star comes out on stage all dressed up and sings one verse: "I'm gonna sing till I die" and then collapses. I yell, "Get me Kidinthechorus!" I rush into Nancy's room. "Do you know the part," I demand. "Do you know the steps? No? I'll teach them to you on the way to the stage."

The show is a flop, but Nancy is a success and becomes a big smash star. I fall on hard times and drop out of the picture. Nancy arrives at a theater all dressed up and surrounded by her retinue.

"I wish we could find Morris," she says wistfully.

"It's not Morris, it's Maurice!" I yell as I reemerge.

"Where have you been?" she asks.

"I've been doing radio in Australia" is the best lie I can come up with.

I get offered one line in her new play: "All you have to say is, 'Dinner is served.' " But I can't get the darn thing right. "Dinner is survived. Dinner is severed. Dinner is serverved." There were a lot of fun songs in the sketch with lyrics such as, "If your best pal and your gal leave you, or both of them deceive you, what do you do — say hello to the moon."

Another hybrid show business parody was "The Dancing Towers," where we married *The Lost Weekend* with dance team movies of the Fred Astaire and Ginger Rogers variety, like *Top Hat, Flying Down to Rio,* and *The Story of Vernon and Irene*

Castle. As a dancer, I was intent on creating new moves and styles. I stumbled onto a new dance style by literally tripping ("I want to start something new. I may not even use my feet!"). Instead of booze, it was food I couldn't get enough of. I kept yelling things like, "Get me a corned beef sandwich, all fat." Every time we danced into a new era, I got fatter.

The first movie I ever saw was in New York City at the Roxy Theater. It was *All Quiet on the Western Front*, with Lew Ayres, one of the most powerful movies about World War I. Seeing a picture like that as a kid and seeing it years later as a man, I had two completely different experiences.

It still holds up as an honest antiwar drama. Ayres plays a German college student during World War I. He is brainwashed into enlisting in the army (along with the rest of his class) by a zealous college professor. On the front lines he quickly discovers that the glory of the Fatherland is of little concern to a soldier dodging bullets and explosions.

The last scene is the film's most powerful. It has Ayres reaching out of his trench for a beautiful butterfly, trying to recapture some sense of humanity among the horrors that surround him, when he gets shot. When we did a satire of the picture, we focused on that last scene. In the film, there is a close-up of the soldier's open, empty hand after he gets shot. It was a powerful scene to show at that moment — it told you what war was all about.

I certainly knew that war was not anything we could make fun of, but I was drawn to the film. I had to study it. War is life magnified a thousand times.

What we ended up scripting was that instead of dying right away, my soldier would keep moving and manipulating his fingers as he dies. One finger moved, another moved, and then my hand was dancing. There was a close-up on my hand, and the audience in the theater got to see it on the big screen over the stage. I actually kept it going for fifteen to twenty seconds. I kept manipulating my hand. I could have gone on for a little longer, but I knew when to stop. Again, we were combining comedy and pathos, working both sides of the street.

I met the director of *All Quiet on the Western Front*, Lewis Milestone, years later in Paris and asked him about the last scene. He said they had staged charge after charge, explosion after explosion. Machine guns had mowed men down by the thousands. They'd already blown up half the world. He wasn't sure how to end the picture. And then he came up with the idea of the butterfly, which was the complete antithesis of war.

Another war movie we were famous for doing was *From Here to Eternity*, the Hollywood version of the James Jones novel, which we called "From Here to Obscurity."

One of the scenes we parodied was the one where Ernest Borgnine pulls a knife on Frank Sinatra and reluctant trumpet player Montgomery Clift breaks a bottle and steps in with the jagged edge. But when my character, whom we named Montgomery Bugle, smashed the bottle against the bar, it doesn't break. I kept banging and banging it against the bar but nothing happens. It was a wooden bottle. I finally said, "I don't need a bottle to rip you apart; I can do it with my bare hands. You're finally showing your true colors — chartreuse."

The part of the film everyone remembers is the classic beach scene with Deborah Kerr and Burt Lancaster, where they are making love on the beach and the waves roll in on them. It was a very passionate scene and for what they were allowed to show at the time, very evocative. It still is. But we saw it and thought, "How can you have sex with the water all over you? It's ridiculous." So we did a takeoff on it.

I was wearing black socks because I didn't have time to take them off during the quick costume change. I was also holding a big inner tube. Immy was in fishnet stockings, and both of us were on a fake beach getting real water splashed on us by the stagehands to simulate the incoming tide during the passionate love scene. The water was supposed to be warm and had probably started out that way. But the stagehands had left the water in the buckets offstage, and you better believe it had gotten pretty cold.

I'd given the crew specific instructions: Take it easy, let us say a line and then throw the water. The guys, however, got a little overzealous. The result was that when Immy and I did the scene, the water was coming so fast we couldn't say the dialogue. The guys kept hitting us in the face and mouth. Every time I opened my mouth, I got a pail of water thrown in my face. I finally ad-libbed, "It's kinda rough tonight!" Immy, who never lost it, cracked up and had to hide her face in my shoulder to keep the audience from seeing her breaking up. The audience wasn't hiding their laughter.

One of the most elaborate movie satires we did was "Aggravation Boulevard," which ran for over forty minutes without any interruptions. It was a takeoff on *Sunset Boulevard*, the Billy Wilder/William Holden/Gloria Swanson classic about an aging silent movie star and her romance with a young screenwriter. Our idea was to build the piece around a male silent icon, the late John Gilbert.

Gilbert, who starred in over a hundred pictures, was one of the biggest names of the silent movie era. He'd been everything from the Count of Monte Cristo to a Latin lover. Greta Garbo had been in love with him and nearly married him. When talkies came, Hollywood legend says his voice recorded very high and that killed his career as a leading man.

The writers and I talked the idea through and I liked it. I became Rex Handsome, the famous silent movie matinee idol, the star of "The Sword of Xarro," "No Man's Land," and "A Doughboy's Heart." Rex is the lead star of Vita-Cash studios, also home to his glamorous actress bride, Mara Bara (Nanette), and producer Flo Floren (Carl), a character we based on legendary producer Florenz Ziegfeld.

I found the voice, several octaves higher than my own, a kind of a whiny voice that was funny and completely unbefitting a great romantic male lead. The sketch started to have legs.

Before I felt comfortable doing the sketch, however, I put in a call to Clara Bow, who was also a legend of the silent movie era. She had been very close to Gilbert. I was very excited about actually calling Clara Bow. I was a great fan of hers and, of course, she had been in the movie *Wings*, the basis for the first sketch Dave and I wrote together, the airplane sketch that helped me become a star.

I told Miss Bow we were going to do a satire on the silent era and the advent of talkies and I wanted to use John Gilbert as the basis for a character to build it around, but that we wouldn't do it without her blessing. She was happy to hear from me, and grateful for the consideration. She thought for a moment and said, "For you, he would have been happy to be a part of it."

"Is Rex Handsome here yet?" Flo asks his assistant at the opening of the sketch. "The front half of his car came through the studio gates twenty minutes ago. He should be here any minute," is the reply.

Announced by his chauffeur (Howie), Rex enters the studio with two Russian wolfhounds, and his adoring director puts him and Mara into the scene. "Now slink over to him," he instructs Mara. "Slink, slink, that's it. Slinkier! Slinkier! Oh, that's fine, you really slunk it up." An underling interrupts the scene with news that talking pictures have just come in. "Rex, do you know what this will do for you?" Flo says. And then the revelation: Rex squeaks, "At last the world will hear me talk! They'll hear Rex Handsome talk. And talk and talk and talk!"

With the advent of talking pictures, the studio switches Rex's latest film, "The Sheik from Oxford," to sound. Because of the changes we made to the Century Theater, we were able to simulate the full effect of a movie premiere. We had a limousine parked at the stage door. We ran out the door, got into the limo, and changed costumes in the car. The limo drove a few dozen feet down to the corner and parked in front of the Century Theater. We had searchlights set up outside and when I got out of the limousine, we had real police officers give us an escort and follow us into the theater. John Gilbert would have been proud.

I get out of the car dressed in a camel

hair coat, again with the Russian wolfhounds. The audience surrounding me was played by actors, singers, and dancers from the *Caesar's Hour* company. We also put people in the lobby of the theater, cheering and screaming. All of a sudden we had a Hollywood opening. And it was all done live.

The elation at the premiere quickly vanishes when Rex speaks on screen in a high-pitched falsetto. The audience howls with laughter at the dashing star with the squeaky, high voice.

Stunned and shunned, Rex sits by the phone for four long years waiting for the studio to call. His house man, also played by Howie in a great takeoff on Erich von Stroheim, calls him daily from across the living room, pretending to be a studio head that Rex then rebuffs in a comically pathetic game.

"Perhaps they've forgotten your number, sir," Howie says.

"Forgotten my number? My telephone number is Crestview One! It's the first telephone number in the world!"

Mara, now a big star with a lot of clout, convinces Flo to offer the despondent Rex a role in her new picture. Rex accepts, and shooting starts on a western. As Rex delivers his first line, the entire set bursts out laughing. Dejected, Rex walks off the set. When he returns, wet from a walk in the rain, he starts speaking in a wonderfully deep voice. Everyone is stunned, and they realize that Rex's voice changed because he caught a cold. Rex heals quickly and he starts talking in his squeaky voice. Mara throws a pitcher of water on Rex and his deep voice returns. Rex will become a film star again, making pictures only when he has a cold.

I always liked the ending to that sketch. The star walks out of the studio in disgrace in the rain, but when he walks back in with the rain at his back he talks with a deep, masculine voice. "Some people in Hollywood are only given one chance," he says at the close. "I was fortunate to be given two. And I know for every broken heart there's an empty swimming pool on Aggravation (his voice breaks into a high pitch, and he throws some water on himself to deepen it again) Boulevard." You can't beat that for a close.

Chapter 13

SENSE MEMORY AND SILENT MOVIES

One skill that came to me naturally is my ability to pantomime. I've always had a good sense memory, which as a performer helped me when we did what was called "in-one sketches." It was just me, performing against the curtain, doing a routine with no scenery and no one to play off of. It is a very pure form of comedy. I peopled the stage and I filled it with scenery. But I was the only one out there.

As with the double-talk, nobody taught me how to pantomime. I learned it myself. It was not always a short, silent pantomime but a combination of mimicry, farce, sense memory, everything. I've been doing it since I was a kid. When I lit a pantomime cigarette, I picked the cigarette up, I held a space for it in between my fingers and was able to remember to give it weight and width for the entirety of the sketch. I could feel the pain that came from dropping cigarette ashes into my open palm. If there was an imaginary dog, I could see the dog in front of me and feel it pulling me or biting my leg. I had always been able to see the props in my mind's eye, and they became real to me. It is a very pure form of theater — it is character and situation driven.

Whenever I did a pain take in any context I never yelled. The secret to the pain take is in not screaming. You internalize the pain. You take a deep breath and your mouth opens and nothing comes out. No noise. Nothing. Your eyes look as if they are going to shoot out of their sockets and fly across the room.

Actors like Robert De Niro, Al Pacino, Harvey Keitel, Robert Duvall, and Dustin Hoffman were trained in the Actor's Studio by Lee Strasberg in what was called sense memory and effective memory. It is a wonderful acting device for arriving at a very private, personal moment, which is perfect for film and television. When you're in the trailer or dressing room and they say, "Okay, come on out, we're ready for you now," you come out and you're ready.

I always said all you really need for a sketch is a table and two chairs. In pantomime, the audience has to work. And they like to work because it's a puzzle to them, and figuring out what is happening is part of the fun. The audience gets to see what is going on in *their* mind's eye.

As desperate as live television was, you usually had somebody to play off of. But in this format, you're out there alone, working a high wire act without a net. And that's when you're most vulnerable. You're standing up there and you're doing a mini-one-man play, with no one to talk to or react against. There was a tremendous level of precision required. You don't have scenes, you don't have costumes, you don't have people you can play off of. There's no rhythm you can tap into, so you have to make your own. You had to remember where you left the first guy and when you shook hands with the other guy, or when you talked to the woman. Once you put the wire up there, you had to stand on it. Then you have to balance yourself, and all the while you're doing your tricks.

You set the audience up and put a picture in their mind. You start with a guy asking his boss for a raise. There are a million variations on that theme and a million things that could be done. But you still have to see the boss there. You have to see his attitude, and the employee's subservience to the boss. If you're walking with someone, you have to remember to put your arm around him or her. The moment you let go or don't pay attention, you fall off the wire, and the audience stops believing you.

One week we were looking for something for me to do in a pantomime sketch. The writers said, "Sid, why don't you pick up a jar of olives and try to open it up but it's stuck." I was doing all kinds of grimaces, making faces. I finally got the lid off. We realized the idea didn't work. So I put the jar down. The writers began to laugh. I said, "What did I do?" They said, "Do you realize you've screwed the pantomime lid back on the jar?"

When I used to do a single, I didn't go out and tell jokes. I used to do situations. Like taking the family out for a Sunday drive. Nobody was there but the chair and me. And I'd say, "No, I didn't forget the soda — it's in the back. Yes, with the sandwiches. And the hot water. No, don't put your hand — I'm driving now. Edward, sit down! Lillian, don't move. John, come over here and sit down. Make room for each other! Johnny, Johnny, get down from that tree! Put the eagle down! Don't play with the eagle!" It was just a family out for a Sunday drive. And it was all sense memory.

I really observed people and tried to duplicate them because people are more interesting than things. Once you capture the people, the audience is involved in the concept. They see the wife, the kids, and the car. I have also been a Russian miner, a French general, a woman getting dressed in the morning, a prizefight manager, a lion in the zoo, a Parisian perfume salesman, a British colonel, a boxer, a cowboy, a gangster, and a doctor. Often the only prop I used was a chair. I did pieces of a guy falling asleep, or trying to go to sleep. Besides the guy asking his boss for a raise, there was a guy telling his mother that he's going to get married (he yells, "Hey Ma, take your head out of the oven") and another going on his first date.

I played a shy boy at his first dance, awkwardly trying to ask a girl to dance, with, much to his embarrassment, his tongue falling out of his mouth and wagging. (That was the time I took on the censors.) The boys stood on one side of the high school gym and the girls stood on the other. The middle was no-man's-land. I then played the same boy five years later, cocky and confident, grabbing a girl to dance, spinning her around, over my shoulders, under my legs, throwing her up to the rafters and catching her.

I was also the husband who has a fight with his wife and then starts to think about all of the things he should've said in the argument. I also played a husband who shows up at a friend's apartment to spend the night after an argument with his wife. I walk on quietly and then start yelling: "Finished! Finished, I tell you. Through. This is the end." I agree that my wife is a sweet and wonderful girl, warm and considerate and everything a man would want. And then I screw up my face in anger and rage. "She's miserable!" I then recount all of my indignities and problems with her. But when she phones to apologize at the end of the monologue, I calm down and go home.

I was a vain man who passes a mirror and is transfixed. I was a reluctant husband being dragged by my wife to a cocktail party. I was also a bridegroom walking down the aisle and thinking pessimistically about my life as a married man. I was an expectant father pacing the maternity ward, thinking about what my son is going to be like and picturing him as a brat and a monster. At seventeen or eighteen he'll come to me and I'll say, "What do you mean you want the keys to the car?" I stand up on my toes and hand him the keys and tell him to be careful as I watch him leave the house. I did that sketch prophetically in 1951 not long before my own son was born. He grew up to be six feet eleven and a doctor.

In another sketch, I'm on the phone with my boss trying to direct him to my house. "Haven't you followed the directions? Go down to Meadowlark Lane, down to the second freeway, and get off at exit 10." He calls back a little while later. "Where are you now?" I give him more directions. It seems I have gotten him hopelessly lost because when he calls again, I say, "Where are you now? . . . they've got to let you back into the country. You're an American citizen!"

I did okay with things as well as people. I was able to play a dial telephone, a slot machine, an elevator, a punching bag, a train, a pool ball, a herd of horses, a tom-tom, a rattlesnake, an infantry battle, a cattle stampede, and a seltzer bottle.

We even humanized a whitewall tire, a right rear tire to be specific. "I just came out of the factory and I'm going to be on a big limousine. I'm going to make new friends. Look where we're going, to all the finest places." I get washed and checked every day. I even make friends with the left rear tire. We go to the finest restaurants and the opera. I was never backed into the curb. I was washed twice a day. It was like that for years.

Then one day everything changes. There is a new owner. All of a sudden I don't get washed every day. No more fancy places. I get banged against the curb. I get loaded down. I'm not going to the Stork Club or to the opera. The limo becomes a cab that goes up to the mountains. We start climbing the mountains and drive faster and faster.

My buddy, the left rear tire says, "Mac, I can't hold out anymore. What's it all about anyway?" I say, "You gotta hold out, for me, you can't leave me now. You can't leave me alone. Who will I to talk to?" But he's too far gone, and one day he explodes. They take him off the rim and throw him on the side of the road, and they put the spare tire on. A new tire that was stuck in the trunk. I've never seen him before.

The new guy is all excited about getting out of the trunk and experiencing new things and new places. "Hey, this is great," the new tire says. I look at him. "You can't even know," I say. "What a life we had." I didn't think I'd miss my old friend, but I really do. I can't get the attention of the front guys; they're too busy steering. And then I get depressed, too. All my friends are gone. I feel myself wearing down. Hold on, buddy, I tell myself. I finally wear down and explode. I blow. They take me off the car and leave me on the side of the road. I lie there in the rain and the mud.

All of a sudden two kids find me and start to roll me. They take me to their backyard. They put a rope on me and I become a swing. It's not bad. I'm in the country and I'm a swing. Fresh air instead of the smell of exhaust fumes. And the kid talks to me all the time. This is a good life. It didn't look like it would be, but it is. I'll be here for years. It was a wonderful metaphor for the life cycle.

These sketches allowed us to reminisce poignantly about the cycles of life and portray them without being melodramatic or maudlin. If we were doing the same sketches with people, they would have been too sad. Investing inanimate objects with life allowed us to do comedy with pathos once again.

Not all of these sketches were solo performances. Immy enjoyed pantomime as much as I, and we did many routines together. We were lions in the zoo and two people fighting over a seat on the subway. On a day at Coney Island, we would eat hot dogs, popcorn, cotton candy, and then go on the roller coaster and try to hold the food down.

We did another pantomime set at a cocktail party. It is just the two of us. I take off my coat and scarf, my hat, and pull my sweater over my head, unzipping and unbuttoning everything. I smile at a beautiful woman and ask her to dance. I take an hors d'oeuvre from a waiter's tray. It has a very bad taste. How am I going to get rid of it? I put it in my hand and shake hands with an imaginary guest, handing it off.

Several of the most memorable pantomimes involved music. One was with Immy doing a pantomime to the *1812 Overture*, playing the instruments and then loading shells for the grand finale. We pinned medals on each other's chests when it was over; we'd earned them. Another was with Nanette. It was an argument set to the music of Beethoven's *Fifth Symphony*. One afternoon, while listening to the *Fifth Symphony* in my office, I thought to myself: "This is an argument!" Nanette and I choreographed the piece as a husband and wife arguing. The two of us go at it, she accuses me of straying after she finds a single long blond hair on me. The payoff to the sketch comes when she learns that the stray hair belongs to our beloved family dog.

In "The Sunday Salon" we are all dressed in white tie and tails for a high-brow concert in a mansion. I come in late with squeaky shoes and sit down. Every move I make has a loud, exaggerated noise. I apologize profusely, showing Imogene that my pocket watch stopped. Winding the watch is extremely loud. Turning on the chair is extremely noisy. Cracking my knuckles sounds like firecrackers going off. I touch my nose and it makes a cracking sound. I ask Imogene what the name of the song is, and I write it down. The pencil touching the paper is very noisy. Tapping my forehead and shaking my head results in a loud tapping sound. I move my toe and it makes a squeak. I close my cigarette case on my fingers and hold it in until I run out into the hall to scream in pain. And then I try to light a cigarette with a gun lighter. As I fire it, Howie falls off his chair. These music sketches were a lot of fun for me.

The longest, most elaborate pantomimes we did involved silent films. A lot of people in our audience remembered silent films and loved them. Before the talkies, the silents used to be great. It's analogous to the way your mother's cooking was the best cooking in the world when you were growing up. That's what silents were to the older audience.

The silent movie sketches were particularly difficult and challenging. We shot them with six cameras, one of which was focused on the cards that showed the viewers the dialogue so they could follow the story. To time these, I told the director to read each card to himself twice before he went to the next shot. When the control room cut to the cards, we couldn't stop acting because we were playing to a live studio audience. Both the crew and the actors needed to be timed perfectly so when the cameras came back to the performance, everyone knew where they were supposed to be and what they were doing.

Many times one or more of the cameras went out. We had to follow the camera that had the red light on it. If a camera went out, it had to be moved off the floor right away and we had to change the choreography immediately. Other cameramen had to cross over in order to set up their shots. We had tech guys whose only job was to keep the cables straight, so that they wouldn't tangle up with each other as the cameras were moved around.

One of our earliest silent movie parodies was of George Bernard Shaw's *Pygmalion*, before it became *My Fair Lady*. Instead of words, we used movements. And we had Charlton Heston, who was a guest a couple of times. He was a very good straight man. He fit in very well.

It was nineteenth-century England, so we all wore top hats, white scarves, and black capes. I was the Professor and Heston played a young gentleman who brings me Immy, a cockney girl who was selling flowers, to teach her how to talk like a lady. I teach her how to sit, how to hold a cup. She keeps putting on her hat, and I keep taking it off. I have her taken upstairs, bathed, and dressed in beautiful new clothes. The moment she comes down the stairs, I instantly fall in love with her. I am smitten — and she spits on me! I get up and start to walk away from her. She runs to my side. "I was only playing a part. I am in love with you."

"A Drunk There Was," which was based on *Stella Dallas*, was the most ambitious silent movie we ever did. It was twenty-eight minutes long and had four scenes. We tried to stretch every creative limit in all of the silent movies and so we made it very realistic in its presentation. The technology didn't yet exist to create the silent movie "iris" effect on the TV screen. We tried a piece of black cardboard over the camera lens to simulate it. It didn't work. So we got a special camera with an iris effect to open and close every scene, to give it authenticity.

I played a man who succumbs to the effects of alcohol, or, as we called it, "demon rum." I start out as a happily married man with Nanette as my wife. It's my birthday, her birthday, our anniversary, and she's pregnant. And the cat had kittens too. So my boss, played by Howie, gives me a raise and proposes a toast to congratulate me. I am now making $6 a week. I don't drink, but I have one at his insistence. "Just one shot," he says. Little does he know that this will be the shot heard round the world. I drink it all down and eat the glass as well. I keep drinking. I'm instantly hooked. My drinking affects my job as a stamp licker. I come in to the office the next morning not well balanced. I have liquor hidden in an inkwell, a flower vase, the bowl of a kerosene lamp, the hollow leg of my desk, and the typewriter roller. Having consumed too much liquor, I try to lick a stamp and miss, and it winds up on Howie's forehead. I am fired by Howie, who is "a friend of the family but an enemy of the bottle." On my way out, I stop at a hat rack, remove the antlers, and drink from the stem.

Our daughter grows up and Carl plays her high-class suitor. "All doors were open to him," reads the title card, "because of his high school diploma." The scene cuts to the outside of a mansion in the rain, as I tearfully watch my daughter get married. Howie raises the shade and waves to me as a cop pushes me to move on. "An ounce of love is worth a case of scotch," is the moral of the story that flashes on the screen. At the end of the sketch, still in my water-soaked costume, I got on camera and told the viewers and the studio audience that "the movie was done in the spirit of good fun" and added that we hoped they got something out of the moral. A mea culpa was needed; it was important that we were clear that we weren't making fun of alcoholics. What the audience and the world didn't know was that I had a drinking problem of my own at the time.

We followed that intensely dramatic piece and closed the show with an installment of the Haircuts. We got cheers the moment we walked on stage. I introduced Carl, Howie, and myself as the brothers: Stacey, Stushee, and Stayshee Haircut. We sang "Only You" in our new "Zephyr sound." I did my best soprano, Rex Handsome voice.

We were just jumping around on the stage, drained from the earlier "A Drunk There Was" sketch. It offered an important counterbalance.

Chapter 14

THE PERILS OF LIVE TELEVISION

I once gave a lecture about comedy at Columbia University. The audience not only had students but also professional writers, producers, directors, and actors, including ones that had shows on the air. When I finished the lecture, we opened the floor to questions. A young television producer raised his hand. "Mr. Caesar, we understand that the show was ninety minutes long, and it was done live. But could you tell us how long did it take to shoot the hour and a half?"

I looked at him and I said, "About ninety minutes. Ninety minutes was it." He wrote it down. He followed up with another question: "Well, what — what did you — if something didn't get a laugh what did you do?" I said, "We went a little faster." He wrote that down too and said thank-you.

People today have no idea what live television means. Doing it live changes the performance equation. Live is a different animal. Live TV was both euphoric and horrifying, a combination of theater and television that was challenging, demanding, and amazingly rewarding. It was flying by the seat of your pants for an hour and a half. In some ways, the only similarity between television today and what we did fifty years ago is that both are watched from a box in people's living rooms.

Live meant no cue cards, no TelePrompTers, no second chances, and no net. You only had one shot — one chance and that's it. If a fly landed on your nose, you squinted and you kept walking and talking and doing the scene, or you incorporated the fly into the scene. The show went on at nine o'clock Saturday night, ready or not. If we ran over, the network would slice us off in the middle of a sentence and the audience would be watching the next program in the schedule. That actually happened once.

In live television, you were your own editor. There were no pickups, dubbing, or fixing mistakes. You needed to feel the audience. Your antenna had to be out for every performance. You had to know when you were winning them over. We would play off each other and work pieces of business. But no matter where I took a piece, I always came back to the cue. You never left a fellow performer hanging out there. When you work live and you go out in front of the audience, you need to be constantly prepared. Your adrenaline has to be up to the performance level. You need to feel the audience so you know how far to go with a piece of business or an ad-lib. That doesn't happen when you do it in bits and pieces. You lose the continuity and the spontaneity. Live, if something happens, you wing it.

When we were doing our shows, television didn't come wrapped as a neat little package with a neat little ribbon. Today, series run for roughly twenty episodes a season and they're all on tape. Today the mentality is, "Let's take it again." You couldn't do that back then. You don't even have to laugh today. They have machines that laugh for you.

The laugh track hurt television comedy more than it helped it. The laugh track laughter became a fixture, like wallpaper. Nothing fails. Everything gets a laugh. But if everything gets a laugh, then nothing is funny.

I think what has happened to comedy between the great days of live television and now is that there are too many people between the comedian and the audience.

In the live days, you couldn't be edited. If you felt the rhythm of the audience you could keep them entertained. No one could change it. Now, by the eighth take, it's not that fresh anymore. Ideally, comedy should be very pure with no one between the performer and the audience other than the cameraman. Now it all comes packaged and a lot of the humanity is lost.

Think about professional sports. Would you rather watch a football game live or on tape? In live television, there is more opportunity to see the humanity of the situation. How exciting would the game be if it weren't live? How many people would sit down to watch a game if they knew how it was going to end and how each play would turn out? There's a big difference between taped and live television. In live television, as you say it, it goes out to the world.

Because of the networks and the advertisers, we have gone from a fifty-three-minute hour to a thirty-eight-minute hour for network television. Now even the Super Bowl is an exercise of not letting the football get in the way of the commercials. Last year, after eight minutes of commercials, I forgot where the game was.

On *Your Show of Shows*, we had three commercial breaks in a half hour (as opposed to

11 commercial minutes in today's half hour). Commercials were read live on the air and each commercial was a minute and ten seconds long. During the extremely brief time between the director yelling, "Into commercial!" and, seconds later, "Out of commercial!" we had to do costume and scene changes. One minute and ten seconds. Think of it. When you heard the words, "Into commercial!" you moved fast to get your costume changed, sometimes in front of the audience with the dressers covering you with a blanket or a sheet. And when you heard "Out of commercial!" ready or not, you were moving back into the show.

Because there were so many places to fail, success was ten times as sweet in live television. No matter how hard you tried, things didn't go exactly as planned. No matter what happened — and did things ever happen — you had to handle it. You couldn't freeze. You had to deal with whatever came your way. It's called thinking. You came up with something right there. Sometimes it got a laugh and sometimes it didn't. But that's all part of the game. You had to make do with what you got. You had to know how to ad-lib. Everything had to be taken in stride.

One of my worst experiences occurred when Max changed the running order at the last minute and switched two sketches. It was quick and confusing. I looked at my dresser. "Mark, did you get that?" "Don't give it another thought, Mr. Caesar — it's all written down. All taken care of." As it turned out, not quite. I went upstairs and prepared to be the strong man in the circus. I was in leotards with a leopard skin loincloth, gold lamé boots, armlets, and a wig. I looked out on stage and saw Carl sitting on a bench, ready for a sketch about two businessmen waiting for a bus.

It was a surreal moment. I felt like it was a dream — actually a nightmare — and I was going to wake up any second. Because you're almost on the air, dressed for the wrong role, you only get about a second and a half to panic. After that you have to channel that energy into action. I started improvising, yelling: "Pants, shirt, coat! Pants, shirt, coat!" Pulling one stagehand over and taking his coat, I took someone else's shirt and pants, grabbed a hat from someone else. I didn't button anything. It was frenetic.

I put the hat on and walk out onto the stage. Carl is sitting on the bench. "Oh, there you are," he says in character.

"Kinda late today, how are you?" "Oh just fine, just fine. I had trouble dressing this morning." And I sat down on the bench and unconsciously crossed my legs and you see these gold lamé boots sticking out there. Without missing a beat Carl said, "Wow, those are great boots. Where did you get them?" I look at him and I put my foot up and say, "Everyone in Rome is wearing them these days. They may look nice, yeah, but they're a lot of trouble. You've got to shave them in the morning, you've got to feed them at night — it gets to be a real pain."

There were other times when we got word from NBC executives that the network had decided to run past the half hour by two minutes, so that the viewers wouldn't change the channel during a commercial break. I would watch for signals onstage and immediately start ad-libbing to stretch out a piece. It was tremendous pressure.

One night during a very successful show, I was doing a monologue about an argument with my wife. "You want the last word? You got the last word. You got it, I love you." I was almost ready to bow. And I look off camera and I see the stage director near the cameraman giving me the hand gestures to stretch the sketch. Immediately

I dive in one more time. "You gonna start again? I'll tell you what. Let's open up the window; let's let the neighbors hear. My wife is now going to make a speech because she's never been heard in the neighborhood." I ad-libbed this whole thing, and then finally I got the signal that we were out of time and I said, "You don't want to talk, then don't talk."

Because of our popularity, the top celebrities in the country wanted to be guests on the show. The problem was, movie stars were generally terrified of live television. They were very interesting people and very talented people, and they all had one thing in common: they weren't used to the one-take format. They were used to three, four, five, or six takes. All of a sudden they found out that they had less than a week to learn all of the lines and sketches and that they had to do it live — one shot. And no cue cards to boot.

A lot of the stars' agents didn't appreciate the differences between the movies and live television. The truth was, it was much more like theater than movies. You can see when somebody else is going to do something because they're looking at you. You have to remember that you have to go and then he's going to come in. You have to wait for the telephone to ring before you can lean towards it. As soon as somebody stops talking, you start talking. Unlike movies, there is always the danger of missing a cue, there is always a distraction. But because it was also terrific exposure for their clients, the agents exposed them to the new medium. Some without warning.

Basil Rathbone, who was in *The Adventures of Robin Hood* and *The Mark of Zorro* and later played Sherlock Holmes, was terrified of live television. Unfortunately I didn't help allay his fears. When I went out to introduce Basil, I said, "Here ladies and gentlemen is . . ." I couldn't believe it, I forgot his name. I had an hour and a half show in my head, and I couldn't remember his name. So I began to stall: "Here is a man whom you've seen play Sherlock Holmes many, many times. He's one of the most experienced theater actors in the world . . ." But I still couldn't think of his name. Finally someone wrote it down on a big piece of cardboard and brought it close enough for me to see it. With great relief, I said, "Mr. Basil Rathbone."

Basil came out and he knew what happened. He was very gracious about it, but he couldn't resist saying, "I'd like to thank

Mr. Sid Silvers for having me on." He got even. I told the director, "Next time, have a card ready with the guest's name on it. Just the name. Just in case."

Another British performer who was a victim of the perils of live television was Sir Cedric Hardwicke. He was a distinguished actor who had played in over eighty movies. He had been King Arthur in *A Connecticut Yankee in King Arthur's Court* as well as the man Spencer Tracy had asked, "Dr. Livingstone, I presume?" Sir Cedric's troubles started with the terrible elevator we had at our theater. It had a heavy door that would swing back hard if you didn't hold it. When he first got out of the elevator, Sir Cedric had let go as he was taking off his hat, which was a derby, and the door swung back at him. It was a good thing he had the hat because that's what got smashed instead of him. We all ran over to help him. He was a very gracious and very elegant man, and he dealt with indignity with much dignity.

He was less lucky on show night. We did a sketch where Sir Cedric played Caesar (not me, the Roman one). There was a slave market, and he was supposed to bid on different slave girls. He came down a sloped staircase with a low ceiling, where you had to duck a little. He forgot to duck and banged his head as he was rushing down. As a result, he was disoriented and had no idea where he was.

Seeing this, I immediately grabbed him and guided him to his mark. I wound up saying all of his lines as well as my own. "This man wants this woman." "Is that true, sire?" "Yes, it is true." You had to do it.

Because I found that some actors tended to read the cue cards instead of playing to their performing partners, I did not allow cue cards or any other form of prompting. I had a hard-and-fast rule. I always said if you are looking somebody straight in the eye, you're acting. Because acting is watching and listening. Good comedy comes from good acting, which is reacting. It's not only the words that are said, it's the way they are being said and your reaction to it. If you are looking at a cue card, you are not looking into someone's eyes, and you can't see the look on their face or their body language, which is going to shape how you reply.

You always knew, for instance, when a colleague forgot a line because their eyes started to widen and you would have to jump in immediately and say something like, "Weren't you expecting a phone call?" And if the person you're playing with says something that you can catch and latch on to, you can make the scene and the sketch funnier.

Even people with small parts sometimes forget. That's what happened when we did a sketch that married legendary attorney Clarence Darrow in *Inherit the Wind* and *The Defenders*, one of the popular TV lawyer shows at the time. Carl played the prosecutor and I played the defense attorney with Howie as my client. I got up and, in my best Lionel Barrymore, I began my closing statement. "How can you convict a man of this caliber? The money he gives to charity. He is a man of the people. He has a wife and children. This man has a life to live; this man has feelings. This man made a mistake. He didn't mean it. Even if he did do it, this man is not guilty. He couldn't have been there. Why would he be sitting there explaining himself? You cannot convict this man. Tell me why, why? You cannot convict this man, please."

The actor that played the foreman got up and said, "Your honor, we didn't have to deliberate for very long. We have come to our decision. The defendant is *not* guilty." He was supposed to say, "We find the defendant guilty."

For a second, I froze. We had half a sketch to go and the thing had suddenly completely changed direction. Mel Tolkin literally screamed from the control room when he heard the mistake.

I jumped in. "What do you mean, not guilty? I'm his defense lawyer. Of course I'm going to say that! I'm telling you with my heart the man is guilty. Understand me when I'm saying, guilty. He's guilty, but I will *prove* to you why he's not guilty." The poor actor wanted to kill himself over it. I made sure he had a part the next week.

Even animals, who didn't have to worry about missing lines, made mistakes on live TV. This happened during one of our Englishmen sketches. The simple premise of these recurring pieces was that Imogene, Carl, Howie, and I would dress up as staid, upper-crust Englishmen and just sit there, unflappable. Nothing was supposed to get to us — in one sketch it poured rain and we wouldn't respond.

This particular sketch used a chimpanzee. During rehearsal the chimp broke up everyone on the crew by walking all over us, even biting my ear. We wouldn't move. It was hysterical. Right before the show, though, the trainer fed the chimp, and during the live broadcast, the chimp just sat there. I had bananas all around me, and in most of my pockets, but the chimp didn't move. We were dying. Max cut the sketch short and Carl and I hastily improvised a Professor interview. I didn't make sure the chimp had a part the next week.

No matter what happened onstage, I never allowed anybody to break up on the show during a sketch. When you laugh during a sketch all of a sudden it becomes an inside joke and the audience feels alienated. The others lost it a few times, and although I came close several times, I never did.

The one incident that really tested our resolve was another Englishmen sketch, this one set in a billiard room where Carl and I were playing pool. We were keeping score and muttering things to each other like "Blackpool for some whitefish, and Whitepool for some blackfish." Each time I used my pool cue, I ripped the felt on the table. The sound effect was like ripped underwear. Carl plunged his cue into the cloth. He tried to remove it. It broke in his hand. This was not part of the sketch. Out of necessity, we began to ad-lib. I picked up a big club and began using it on the table like a polo mallet. Carl kept saying "Good shot!" We kept aiming and shooting and the felt on the table kept ripping, all to great sound effects. Carl tried so hard to keep from breaking up that he bit a hole on the inside of his mouth. He couldn't breathe.

The chaotic nature of live TV meant that teamwork was an integral part of the show. One week I came in at 10:00 a.m. on show day. The union was considering a strike, and the crew had staged a slowdown. The camera guys were going over the shots frame by frame as part of the slowdown.

I could feel the tension among the crew, who were professionals trying to do a great job. Just because the union ordered a slow-down didn't mean they were happy about it. I didn't like the level of frustration that the crew was going through. Good friends were snapping at each other. I didn't want any more of that kind of rehearsal. I saw what was going on, and asked if we could run through the show once.

"You guys know what you're doing? You know where the shots are?" I asked at the end of the run-through. They told me they did. So I canceled the dress rehearsal and sent the crew out for lunch on me and told them to come back at 7:30. During the actual show, out of about five hundred or six hundred shots, they missed two very unimportant shots. They ended the show congratulating each other on how well they did. Comradery and teamwork always went a long way with us.

Live television was especially hard for me because I am a fundamentally shy person, which is probably surprising for someone who has appeared in front of millions of people. That's why I developed a cough, which allowed me time to think and speak. Larry Gelbart wasn't kidding when he said that the hardest thing I had to say was "good evening ladies and gentlemen."

There were times where I felt I was shrinking away. Holding on to the microphone helped. And if I became the character, that was something else to hide behind. You're freer to stretch. Jack Benny and George Burns were doing themselves, but they were also performing a character part that they created.

The best part of being an entertainer is making people laugh. It's an absolute tonic. It's like stepping into air. You can't see that next step but you trust yourself and you take it anyway. And it's there. And if the audience is with you, and the timing is with you, you have control over both the audience and the subject matter.

Nights when we had great shows were

like that. The audience reaction was marvelous. The cast worked exceptionally well together. I would walk offstage into the dressing room literally a few feet off the ground on a cloud of euphoria. The night we did "This Is Your Story" was one of those nights.

By the fourth season of *Your Show of Shows*, Max was taking a full half hour for the operettas, so he let me have my head and really run with a sketch. This one was a parody of the very popular TV show, *This Is Your Life*. It is also one of my all-time favorite sketches because it took amazing amounts of energy and creativity, and is a prime example of comedy with pathos. By this time we'd moved from the International Theater to the 5,000-seat Center Theater, which was on 51st Street and Sixth Avenue, a block north of its sister theater, the Radio City Music Hall. It had revolving and elevated stages that we didn't know what to do with. We didn't have enough chorus girls to fill that stage, although we thought about getting some more.

Because "This Is Your Story" was so physically demanding and exhausting, we never rehearsed the sketch in its entirety. It required too much energy. We saved ourselves for the fifth blocking, which was the actual Saturday night performance. As was often the case, many of the great things we did were invented live onstage.

Carl did a wonderful job as the Ralph Edwards–type host, walking into the audience to find the person whose intimate life story would be told that night. It was the first time cameras were ever turned on the audience on our — or perhaps any — show. I played Al Duncey, an ordinary working stiff who is sitting in the audience minding his own business. Carl gets closer, priming the audience for the person he is going to choose to have the intimate details of his or her life broadcast to millions of people. I am sitting there smugly feeling sorry for whoever the poor soul is going to be. Even when Carl gets to my row, I'm certain he's going to choose the guy sitting next to me (played by an NBC executive named Dave Tebet, who was also Nanette's first husband).

According to the original script, I was supposed to say some dialogue after Carl says, "This is your story, Al Duncey." But when I realize that it's me, I faint. Then, according to the plan, as Carl keeps grabbing at me, I pull away and make the theater a character in the sketch. I run into the aisle and am chased by NBC ushers around the theater and across the stage, ducking, faking, cutting into different directions, trying to escape from the theater. The ushers catch me and literally carry me onto the stage, struggling all the way.

As the show gets going, I hear a series of offstage voices from my past. The first voice says, "Hello, Al. Remember me? I used to encourage you. I helped you during those desperate years . . ." I ask if I can hear it again. And out comes Howie as, who could ever forget him, the irrepressible Uncle Goopy. As Uncle Goopy and Al, Howie and I played it way over the top, hugging each other and crying like there was no tomorrow. Our reunion won't end. We smother each other with hugs and kisses. Each time Uncle Goopy is ushered off into the corner so that another relative or friend can be brought out, we rush back into each other's arms, continuing our effusive reunion. Howie is literally hanging all over me, clinging to my leg as I walk. After he falls to the floor, in one swift moment, I pull him back up by his heels onto the couch and into my arms.

Carl grabs Howie and puts him under his arm, carrying him back to his chair in the corner. Carl was working very hard to keep the show moving, and we were doing our best to keep that from happening. Our repeated embraces showed no signs of calming down and neither did the audience's reaction to the repetition. We just kept feeding off the energy of the audience and were able to run with the bit.

One by one, long-lost folks come out to meet Al, including Aunt Mildred from South Africa and Mr. Torch, a firefighter who once rescued Al from a burning building (who was played by Louis Nye, a funny comedian who was one of Steve Allen's *Tonight Show* regulars).

Now a beautiful woman appears from behind the curtain. I stand up and look at her. "Do you remember me?" she asks. "Oh honey, baby," I say. I start to hug and kiss her. And kiss and kiss. Oh yeah. The kisses start getting passionate. Carl asks, "Do you mind telling us who this is?" I raise my head momentarily and say, "I don't know who she is, but it's alright with me," and I go back to kissing her.

Carl looks into his book and realizes that the woman is a guest for next week's episode of *This Is Your Story*. I couldn't care less and keep pushing him away as I continue kissing the beautiful stranger. The audience is having a great time with it. The last big surprise for Al is a reunion with a group he used to be part of, and the Northern New

Jersey Drum and Bugle Corps marches loudly onto the stage. We all get together on the couch and salute and hug each other.

It was a very emotional sketch because at its core it was about reuniting with loved ones you haven't seen in a while. We mocked the purported reality and the alleged warmth of the show. The beauty of a parody like that is that you don't need to see even one episode of *This Is Your Life* to find the sketch hysterical.

Perhaps the most significant ad-lib I ever did was in "Galipacci," our takeoff on the opera about the sad clown Pagliacci. I was at the dressing room table ready to sing my arioso. I was putting on my makeup right after discovering that I've been cuckolded. I'd just begun looking into the mirror, painting tears under my eyes with a mascara pencil when all of a sudden the point of the pencil broke, leaving a big mark on my face. The writers, watching from the control booth, were terrified; everyone offscreen was holding their breath. Painting tears was no longer an option, but the pencil breaking became a found comedic moment.

When I saw the line on my face, thought, I might as well go through with

I put down the pencil, picked up a little paint brush, and made another vertical line on top of the first one, and then another line, and all of a sudden I started playing tic-tac-toe on my cheek. I'm not just doing x's and o's, I'm actually playing a game out there while I'm singing the arioso in Italian double-talk. I win the game at the same time I sing the final refrain in English, Cole Porter's "Just One of Those Things." I measured the song out with the playing of the game. As I came to the end of the aria, I had three x's. I won. The audience had no idea that it was all ad-libbed. Sometimes it comes to you from nowhere, but thank God it did.

Later that evening, relaxing after the show at Danny's Hideaway, the writers and I were at our regular table when I felt a pair of hands on my shoulders. A very light touch. I turned around, and there standing before me was Marilyn Monroe. I was stupefied. What a wonderful moment — to turn around and see Marilyn Monroe standing at the back of your chair with her hands on your shoulders. I just didn't know what to do.

I jumped up, threw the napkin down, nd asked, "Is there anything I could do you?" I was so close to her, I could smell her perfume and her powder. I was like a teenager with raging hormones.

"No, thanks," she said. "I just came over to congratulate you. I never saw anything like that. When you started to play tic-tac-toe on your face, I screamed. I almost wet my pants. So I tracked you down to this restaurant."

"Thank you," I said, "thank you very, very much." I asked if she wanted anything to eat. I think I offered to buy the restaurant for her. I was effusive. I walked her back to her table, I pulled out her chair, she sat down, and then I sat down. I held her hand and thanked her for her kind words. I shook hands with her and I floated back to my own table.

Sometimes the perils of live television are matched by their rewards.

Part 3
A LEGACY IN COMEDY

Chapter 15

CONQUERING DEMONS
NOW, WAS, AND GONNA BE

Mel Funn (Mel Brooks): How are you feeling, Chief?
Studio Chief (Sid Caesar): I'm all right, except for the constant pain.
Silent Movie, 1975

In 1977 I was standing on a stage in Regina, Canada, doing Neil Simon's *The Last of the Red Hot Lovers*, and I could not remember a line of the script. I'd had momentary lapses before, but nothing like this. For the first time in my life, I was on stage and unable to remember what I was supposed to be doing.

It was the first time drinking compromised my ability as a performer. For nearly three decades my addictions had hurt my family and my friends, but they had never hurt my art. I was probably waiting for that absolute lowest point of my life. As an artist, I had just hit rock bottom.

That night, in a shabby little dressing room off the kitchen of the Hotel Regina, I made a life decision. I walked off the stage into the dressing room, sat down, and looked at myself in the mirror. I took a real good look. I asked myself, "Sid, do you want to live or do you want to die?" It was simple as that. There was no gray area, no maybe, no if, no nothing. "That's it," I said. "I can't. No more." I decided that I was going to live.

I checked into a hospital and went through what they call Canadian withdrawal, which was cold turkey, which turned me into a wild turkey. I was watching the clock tick second after agonizing second. I was taken off all pills and then watched carefully to make sure that I didn't go into convulsions as a result of the barbiturate withdrawal, which can be more deadly than heroin withdrawal. Thank God, I didn't.

A couple of years ago, Showtime presented *Laughter on the 23rd Floor*, Neil Simon's movie adaptation of his stage play based on his experiences on *Your Show of Shows* and *Caesar's Hour*. The movie was a lot darker than the Broadway version and focused more on my addictions. While I very much enjoyed the movie and Nathan

Lane's interpretation of me, the movie didn't explain why my character, Max Prince, took pills and drank to excess.

The reason was simple: I couldn't get to sleep. It was my name out there at the top of the show, and the weight of the entire operation rested on my head. Nobody would get blamed but me if something went wrong. As soon as I hit the pillow every night, a newsreel started going on in my head. I would mentally replay sketches and ideas. My mind was constantly racing, thinking of all the variations and permutations: Maybe we could do it like this? Would it be better like that? Maybe if we do it earlier? This was all night, every night; there was no way I could get any rest. I couldn't turn it off. The only thing that helped me get to sleep was getting drunk. I was what they call a "hurry-up drinker." I had to get drunk by ten o'clock because I had to get to sleep and be up early in the morning.

My compulsive personality was part of what made me a successful artist, but the flip side of that coin was the insecurity that led to the addictions. I had little confidence in myself and was fearful that all the success could be taken away. I watched my father lose his business during the Depression and that became my expectation — I would fail and it was only a matter of time before it happened.

As I have said before, you learn nothing from success. Success leads to bad habits. Achieving success without ever experiencing failure is dangerous. It doesn't provide you with perspective, and it makes you terrified of failure. It's when you have your first bounce that you get a message. Failure teaches you about life. Success without ever tasting failure ultimately teaches you only one thing — how to be a jerk.

From the day I joined the Coast Guard, all the way through *Your Show of Shows* and *Caesar's Hour*, it was one straight shot up. I was successful as a musician, as a solo act, on Broadway, and in the movies. My success came too fast, like a rocket; I never failed at anything. If I had experienced a bump in the road professionally earlier on, I think I would have learned.

At the end of the *Caesar's Hour* run, I was at the top of the mountain, national television. I was performing in front of 60 million people a week, but all I could feel was pressure to maintain the level of success. I was making $1 million a year when $5 bought a steak dinner for two.

I enjoyed the laughs, but I never enjoyed

474

the stature. I never believed enough in myself. I had all the accoutrements of show business success — the chauffeured limousine, the clothes, anything money could buy. What I didn't have was the self-confidence. I kept thinking that someone else was doing it, not me. That there was another power driving my success, and that I had nothing to do with it.

I didn't take credit for anything. I didn't want to. I was afraid. I didn't want to be responsible for my own life. And in the 1950s I was popular enough to get away with a lot of things. I wanted to be good, but I didn't walk into anything thinking I was going to be a star. I was a workingman who wanted to be good at what I did. I wanted to learn.

Though I never took a drink before or during the show, I was prone to excesses. What I would do is drink after a performance. A couple of drinks in the dressing room and then I'd go out and have a couple more and then go home. I never thought it would catch up to me. I thought it was social drinking: "Oh, I had two or three drinks." Three drinks were actually nine drinks. I made all kinds of excuses. "So I drink, so what? What's a couple of drinks?" Before I knew it, it was a bottle a night.

I had big appetites. I was the Cadillac running at full speed using a lot of fuel. I ate big meals and, in the evenings, I washed the food down with anywhere from a quart to a quart and a half of scotch. Fortunately, I was throwing up a lot of the food and with it the alcohol. Otherwise, I doubt I would have survived the self-abuse.

The artistic process is rarely without great pain; sometimes the fire is so hot you can't control it. I created my own pain. If I had to start it over again, I would not have touched a drop of liquor. Drinking made my life ten times harder. Given the choice, I would have found another, healthier outlet. On the other hand, if I'd had the choice of producing the body of work or not drinking, I don't know what I would have chosen. I don't know whether I would have given up the pain if it meant not having the ability and opportunity to create and to inspire and entertain so many people and their families.

Alcoholism among celebrities was much less tolerated than it is today. I was afraid to join AA because I was afraid of being exposed. Although they promised anonymity, I was one of the best-known performers in America and lived in fear of discovery and having the network cancel my show. This made getting help and support very risky.

My writers, my friends, were extremely protective of me. They were more than just colleagues. They were menschen. The best-known story is the one affectionately dubbed "The Coleslaw Caper." One Wednesday night during the run of *Caesar's Hour*, something unexpectedly fell apart and we had to write an entirely new sketch in a single day. Carl and the writers and I went to dinner at a nearby restaurant. "First we'll have a drink," I said, "then we'll eat, and then we'll work." What I didn't say was that I'd been taking a strong sedative at the time.

When the waiter came to take the food order after our drinks, I said, "I'll have fillet of sole . . ." and promptly slumped forward, face first, into a bowl of coleslaw. The writers laughed at first, thinking it was a joke. When they realized that I had passed out, Carl told the others that they had to pretend that this was a skit or else the incident would be in all the papers the next morning.

One of the writers stood over me with a knife in his hand and said, "So, Inspector, this undoubtedly is the murder weapon." Another writer responded, "Let us pray," and they all put their heads down on the table.

This kind of improvisation went on for forty-five minutes, with me out cold and the writers periodically checking to make sure I was still breathing. Finally, as the waiter brought the check to the table, my head popped up and I said, "and shoe-string potatoes," picking up exactly where I had left off when I went down into the coleslaw.

What happened in that Canadian dressing room in 1977 began my healing process, but my life really turned around when I went to Paris in 1979. I was offered a job on a less than stellar picture with Peter Sellers called *The Fiendish Plot of Dr. Fu Man Chu*. I was fifty-seven years old. We were supposed to be there for three months. We were there for six.

Peter Sellers and I had dinner together only once. We talked about Spike Jones. We didn't know what to say to each other even though we both began our careers in sketch comedy. Sellers was very sick. He was dying.

I thought those months away would be helpful. It was going to be all about new people and new things. I was less recogniz-able in Paris than I was in the United

States, and I could walk the streets freely. I had a beautiful suite in a charming hotel, the Victor Hugo on Rue Copernic near the Arc de Triomphe (which became a metaphor for a triumph of my own).

I tried to enjoy Paris to the fullest. I would buy oranges and tomatoes, and big hard rounded seedless rye with a great crust. I had never tasted bread so good in my life. I would eat it with cheese and jambon and wash it down with tea with milk.

One evening, after having a great meal, I started walking down the Champs-Elysées in a very good mood. I lit a big cigar and couldn't have walked more than eighty feet when my mood went from high to low. It just vanished in a puff of cigar smoke. What happened to me in eighty feet? A bad habit that I had practiced for many years. A habit that needed to be broken.

I came to a simple yet powerful conclusion: If you make friends with yourself, you can make friends with other people. You have to smile inside. My road to recovery was long and hard, often harder than the pain of addiction. But I made friends with myself.

I now had Paris and the power of my own voice. I brought a small Sanyo tape recorder to the city with me, planning to spend a lot of time in the museums. Since photographs weren't allowed, I'd describe the paintings into the recorder. I wound up using the recorder in a totally unexpected way for something much more vital to my health. I started talking to myself.

I was Sid and Sidney. Sidney was the kid, the one who thought of the crazy ideas. I couldn't put him out of my life. Sid was the man. I became my own psychiatrist. I would set the mood and tone for the day. I'd say, "Sidney, we're gonna be together twenty-four hours a day. Nobody but you and me. If I'm not gonna have a good time, you're not gonna have a good time. So why don't we make friends? Stop thinking about everything that can go wrong. And let's have some fun here while we're at it. Don't you really want to enjoy your life? Enjoy your food, enjoy the walks. Look around and see what you're living through. It's not a dress rehearsal, it's the show."

From September 22, 1979, through mid–1999, not a day went by when I did not speak to that tape recorder. Ultimately, you can't lie to yourself. I conquered my demons. And boy, was it hard. Pain is something you can make bigger or smaller, and in the final analysis you're alone with your own pain. There were a lot of three steps forward two steps back periods. You learn what is important and what is not important. Once you get all your demons out of the way, you look at life differently. All you have to do is get up and take a walk and life is sweet.

I went to psychiatrists for years and I never took to it. I think it's ultimately a matter of nomenclature. It almost felt like a comedy routine: "Your mother was your father and your sister was your brother, but your mother was your sister and your cousin. And your mother was your father, but your sister was your cousin." I don't believe that a psychiatrist can help anyone who drinks or takes pills. You have to do it yourself.

What it boiled down to is the strength to be able to say, "I don't want to think about it." Thinking negatively is the result of guilt and insecurity. I let go of any guilt that I had due to achieving success and surpassing my father. I realized that my father did the best he could under the circumstances and conditions of his life. I made my own luck and my own success. I told myself, "You are the person who makes yourself happy. You're the one who makes yourself sad." It's much easier to feel better when you keep remembering that. I know it sounds very simple and reductive, but sometimes the simple thoughts in life are the most meaningful. We have to stop hiding things from ourselves.

In the early 1980s, while traveling through Kentucky, I came across a beautiful river and noticed that it branched off into two tributaries. The tributary on the right was going to be utilized commercially; the one on the left was flowing tranquilly and naturally. The water on the right was going to work. Industry, growth, production, things people need were all coming out the flowing water on the right side. The water on the left was just rolling along. The image of the river became a metaphor for me. As the waters of your own rivers flow downstream, they can go one way or another, toward productivity or peace, depending on your choices and your time in life.

This — productivity and peace — became a mantra for living my life. I learned how to deal with my fears and insecurities. Once you talk about something and the heavens don't split, you're okay.

If you can control your attitude, you can control your life. Believe that you deserve a little time and a little love. I can't make the point emphatically enough. I never stopped to smell the roses. I never even saw the roses. All I knew was work. I was a driven, quality-obsessed workaholic who was never good at compromise. Now I have a great sense of wonderment about life. I can see roses where most others can't. I now look at the world in a different, healthier way. I think about the flowing water a lot in my day-to-day life.

The most important lesson about both art and life is that you can't do it alone. No one does anything well alone. One of the ways you get through any adversity is with the help of good friends. For me, Rudy DeLuca is one of those friends. Rudy is a very funny comedic actor, writer, and director. People know him best for his work on *The Carol Burnett Show*, where he was Barry Levinson's writing partner for many years, and for collaborating with Mel Brooks on movies like *History of the World: Part One* and *Life Stinks*, as both an actor and a writer.

I met Rudy on the set of *Pink Lady and Jeff*, a short-lived television show that paired comedian Jeff Altman with two beautiful Japanese singers who did not speak a word of English. I played the father to the girls, instructing them (in Japanese double-talk) how to date and threatening their dates with a Samurai sword. I threw some Yiddishisms in, made references to things like being late for temple, and did a James Cagney impression with a Japanese accent. Rudy directed one of the episodes I was in; we connected, and soon we became close friends. We "sparked" each other with ideas and would genially "top" each other with witty comments.

Almost every Thursday for twenty years, Rudy hosted a party. Forty weeks a year, that made for about eight hundred parties. Rudy would go shopping and cook for each event like it was a royal wedding. He would buy and lug fruit home and then meticulously cut pineapples, papayas, and exotic fruit into a salad. There was also a lot of Chinese food. Rudy would never repeat a meal from week to week.

We had a handful of people in our core group, including Corinne Calvet, Dick Shawn, John Byner, Robin Riker, Bill Haisley, Paul and Terry Lichtman, and Charlie Fleischer, a wonderful comedian who's still probably most famous for being the voice of Roger Rabbit. If Rudy invited more than ten people, I would tell him that it felt too much like a cocktail party as opposed to a gathering of friends.

The parties were not only a safe haven

but also a tremendous support system. I learned to laugh again, and laugh hard. With no prior planning, we could lapse into lengthy, intense discussions of specific topics: the two World Wars, France, Russia, the legions of Rome, quantum physics were all acceptable topics of discussion, with a lot of jokes in between. I could say things and try things that I would never do onstage or on television. I could build a bit over why people do what they do, like why someone would have a facial tic. My thoughts went to all kinds of places, and my imagination and creativity ran wild in that safe and creative environment. There was a lot of intellectual and emotional energy that fueled the group. There was an aura about the place and chemistry about the people. There was only one ground rule: You couldn't talk about work or where your career was going.

I needed those parties badly during the valleys, the low points in my career. At meetings with twenty-six-year-old network executives, I would show them "Aggravation Boulevard" and explain how it was done live, pointing out the intricacies of the set and costume changes. The general response would be "so what."

The magic and the artistry of live television was lost on these people. They were also scared by black-and-white. Network executives referred to my comedy as "old comedy." I never thought of comedy as old or new. I always thought of comedy as good or bad. If it makes you laugh, it's good comedy.

One thing I know for sure: If it were not for Florence I would not be alive. I cannot say that emphatically or passionately enough. She stood by me through all my troubles and everything else. Her patience and endurance got me through every bad experience. Florence stuck it out when I was up to a fifth or a fifth and a half of scotch a day. With that I was taking as many as four Equinol and four barbiturates every day. During the toughest times, she flew all over the world and got me out of hospitals. She stayed with me because she loved me.

When I would come home drunk, I wasn't such a nice guy, but Florence would put me to bed. I'd wake up in the morning and she would say, "You know how many people you have to apologize to?" I never saw my house, my gardens, my children — they'd be sleeping by the time I got home at night, or in school when I woke up in the morning, or trying to hide the pills and the bottles from me when I was gone. I did not get to see my kids grow up. I did not get to make peace with them until much later on.

When we lived on Park Avenue I came home one night with a gift for Florence, a beautiful diamond necklace. I had a lot of stuff on my mind that night, so I didn't give it to her with a lot of feeling. She opened it up, looked at it, and threw it back in my face. "When you give something, even if it's a flower or a box of candy, you should do it nicely, do it with some feeling," she said. "It's a marriage, Sidney."

Whenever I am asked what advice I would have given to a John Belushi or a Chris Farley, it would be to find a woman like Florence who would help them through the rough spots. You have to have a solid base to have a strong career and a good life. Florence gave me that support. I cherish my wife as the most important thing in my life. Together, we've done it all.

I appreciate my memories with Florence. They embolden me and make me smile. For instance, there was a tiny bridge over a little stream at Avon Lodge. In the winter, ice would form around it. I think of the times I held Florence on that bridge and just kissed her. Just holding her is one of the best memories of my life.

Other times, I would walk around behind the hotel in the deep woods. There was a certain spot where the sun shone brightly through the trees. After I stood motionless twenty minutes, all the little animals and birds would get used to me and resume their activities. If you don't move, they're there for your entertainment.

As painful as my addictions have been, they would have been even more painful had I not learned anything from them, but fortunately I have. First, you can get away with treating many things lightly in your life but your health is not one of them. As religiously as I drank and took pills, that's how religiously I gave them up. I used my addictive personality and channeled it toward diet and exercise. I even came out with my own exercise video.

Health cannot necessarily be taught; you need self-control and discipline. You need both diet and exercise in your life. If you exercise without dieting, you'll have hard fat. If you diet without exercise, you'll have lean flab. I used to look forward to cigars, which I had after brunch every Sunday. I enjoy just looking at the cigars now.

I still continue a Sunday brunch tradition with family and friends that my brother Dave started with an omelet of his invention. Almost every Sunday, I take twenty-two eggs and I take out all but two yolks. I use only virgin olive oil; I chop up onions, red and yellow peppers, and cook them until they caramelize. When you fry onions and peppers together it gives the omelet a different taste. I add the egg batter in, a little garlic, basil, oregano, and a touch of hot cayenne pepper for a little zip. When it is almost done, I put a plate on top and turn off the heat and let it cook itself. I make the omelets in a large skillet that was given to me by Buddy Hackett, a frequent guest at the brunches.

I don't profess to have all the secrets of how to live life, but I have learned a few things. I respect tradition and history. I study history and I believe in the lessons it teaches. It helps me remember who I am, where I come from, and where I'm going. I am still intellectually curious, still learning and growing. I revel in the moment and appreciate the beauty of nature. I listen to the mockingbirds sing to each other outside of my home. I believe that if you want to do something and it doesn't hurt yourself or anyone else, do it.

I also appreciate my friendships. I have a biweekly lunch with a group of writers and comedians who collectively created some of the greatest comedy of the twentieth century. We share a common history and experience. Each of us understands what the other is talking about. We consistently make each other laugh.

After more than two decades of being alcohol free, I know I'll never go back. My life and my perspective have changed. It took me a long time to be comfortable in my own skin. I spent too many years turning each accomplishment into another reason to be fearful and anxious about the future. To me, artistic success went hand in hand with a self-destructiveness that took its toll on my family, friends, and health, and nearly killed me.

The good news is that I beat my demons. I learned how to enjoy every day, revel in my successes, and not punish myself and the people around me. I went from self-destructive to self-affirming, to being someone who celebrates life instead of someone who constantly fears it, or at least is troubled by it. I still get angry, but I never get as angry as I used to. There is strength and hope and, as simple as it sounds, I enjoy my life. I've achieved a sense of peace, and I am alive to talk about it.

I also relied on the wisdom of Albert Einstein. His theory of relativity is not only applicable to physics, but to human beings as well. Life is too complicated to envision because life, like everything else, is relative. Life is something you have to accept as is. There is no up or down. It's life. You're the one who makes it go up or down. It's not what happens to you in your life; it's what goes on in your head.

I have adopted a very simple philosophy of life. It's called living in the now. What is a now? This is a now. How important is a now? A now goes by at the speed of light, 186,000 miles per second. Einstein said if you wanted to put the special theory of relativity into one sentence, it would be, "One man's now is another man's was." This now is now gone, and we'll never get it back. So how do you live in it if it's gone before it comes? You think about the gonna be.

There's a now, a was, and a gonna be. Now is now, and after now is a was. And what comes after the was is a gonna be. It hasn't happened yet. It's gonna happen as soon as the now is over. But if you have a good now, you're bound to have a good was and a good gonna be. But after the bad now comes a bad was. But if you have a bad now and you dwell on it, you're going to have a bad gonna be and you're going to have a bad cycle. If you learn from the bad was, you can turn the bad gonna be into a good gonna be. The only way you can change the cycle is after the was. If you carry the bad wases around with you, they get heavy and become should'a could'as — I should'a done this, I could'a done that.

If you learn from the was, you'll have a great now; you won't repeat the same mistakes. It will bring you to a good now, which changes the cycle to a good was, and a good gonna be. You need to learn from the wases. It's all about changing your attitude.

We're all moving; we're all getting older. It's not about getting there, it's about enjoying the trip. We can either say we're all slowly dying, or we can say that we're all slowly living. It may be a physical certainty that we are all going to die, but now isn't the time to die. Now is the time to live.

Chapter 16

TEN FROM MY LATER YEARS, AND ONE TO GROW ON

My career after the golden decade of the 1950s was not as frenetic as my *Show of Shows* and *Caesar's Hour* years — how could it be? The next stage of my career was not marked by a week-to-week life but by short-term projects. I did a number of movies, plays, and TV specials that I am especially proud of.

It's a Mad, Mad, Mad, Mad World

It's a Mad, Mad, Mad, Mad World (1963) might have been the first successful big-budget Hollywood comedy. Imagine sitting around with eighteen of the top comedians and comedic actors in the world every morning waiting for the sun to come up to start shooting — people like Milton Berle, William Demarest, Jimmy Durante, Buddy Hackett, Buster Keaton, Ethel Merman,

Carl Reiner, Mickey Rooney, Dick Shawn, Phil Silvers, Terry Thomas, Jonathan Winters, and many others. Even Jack Benny had a drive by. Every comedian in Hollywood wanted to be a part of the picture.

My part in the film had to get done first because I also had a Broadway show and a TV show I was working on. The William Morris Agency got tired just watching me work. They really knew how to book. Fred Allen once said, you could put the heart of an agent in the navel of a flea and still have room for William Morris. I can use that joke because William Morris still does great work for me.

As you can imagine, this was no small production. Filming was supposed to take three months, but it took six. Screenwriter Bill Rose had to turn out two scripts: one for dialogue and one for physical business. Each one was the size of a telephone book.

The story involves a group of strangers accidentally getting together in a frantic search for the hidden money from a bank robbery. There's a big scene in the beginning of the picture where we all pull our cars over to the side of the road to discuss how we're going to split the money that Jimmy Durante's character told us about before he died. I tell the group, "Let's

494

divide up the treasure mathematically. Everyone with one car gets one point . . ."

I had the long speech in that scene; everyone else's dialogue consisted of interruptions. Director Stanley Kramer insisted that we do the entire scene in one master take, so that he could cut in and out whenever he wanted. It was a very intricate scene, with interruptions everywhere. Everything had to be done at exactly the right moment. We finished the day's shooting and Stanley said, "Don't print anything." When a director says don't print anything, that's not a good sign. It can only mean one thing: It didn't go well.

I suggested that the group get together that night in the hotel dining room to work through the scene. We discussed the scene, and though I never acted as the leader, I did give the group the benefit of sketch comedy experience.

The next morning we were out on location at 8:00 a.m. We did the entire scene in one take. Stanley was ecstatic. "What are we going to do for the rest of the day?" he asked, tongue in cheek. Not that he was really worried.

Edie Adams, who played my wife, was a great person as well as a pleasure to work with. Her real-life husband, Ernie Kovacs, a true comedic genius, went much too soon. In one scene Edie and I were trapped in a hardware store. I had a sixteen-pound sledgehammer and was supposed to try to bust down an impenetrable steel door. The grips bet me that I couldn't break the door down. After five shots with the sledgehammer, I knocked the door down. They had to reinforce the sides of the door with more steel for the actual shooting.

Except for scenes that were shot indoors in a warehouse, the movie was shot outdoors. We worked in the 120-degree Palm Springs heat from 8:00 a.m. to 6:00 p.m. Each shot took a long time because of the size of the cast. After each shot, we all needed to have new makeup applied. Even though it was very tiring, everyone was a consummate professional. Today if three comedians get together for a movie, they declare a national holiday.

In addition to working with Buster Keaton, I also got to work with another one of my idols, Spencer Tracy, who played the detective who kept an eye on us. Seeing him made me flash back to the Loews Proctor theater in Yonkers when I saw him on the big screen in *Captains Courageous* with Freddie Bartholomew.

Tracy kept to himself for most of the

shooting. Every morning he would say, "Hello, Mr. Caesar," but we hardly ever spoke. I did have lunch with him and Stanley Kramer in the commissary a few times. I remember the waiter asked, "What will you have, Mr. Caesar?" I pointed to Spencer Tracy. "Whatever he's having," I said.

Tracy was from the old school, which was a very good school. He used to say, "Say the words and don't bump into the furniture." In his day, you walked onto the set and you knew your lines and were ready to go. They didn't take five or six months to shoot a picture. A month was considered a long shooting schedule. The B pictures were shot in ten days.

We got to the set one day and heard that Marilyn Monroe had died. Tracy was really broken up about that. He turned to me and said, "You think they would have stopped shooting for a minute out of respect. A star dies, and the studio doesn't stop for a minute. Clark Gable brought so much money into MGM and no one stopped when he died. There was no respect."

Tracy was sick at the time and negotiated a limited schedule. There was a clause in his contract that he would not work past 4:00 p.m., and every day we'd look for the

Rolls Royce driving onto the set. In the car was the late, great Katharine Hepburn, who would show up at four sharp to pick him up and drive him away. She never got out of the car. I was supposed to do a scene with Tracy and I was really looking forward to it. But when the day came, it was slow shooting. Four o'clock came, and he was gone, and with him went our scene.

When the film finally finished, I got drunk at the wrap party and William Demarest approached me. Bill was a wonderful man, a great actor, and a good straight man, someone who was in practically every one of Preston Sturges's movies.

"Mr. Caesar," he said, "you should sit down and take it easy. People look up to you. They love you. You should have more respect for yourself." He was right. I had a similar response to seeing Judy Garland years later, wanting to be protective when I saw her drinking. Her hat was askew and she had trouble with her lipstick. Even the people with her didn't pay attention to her condition.

Little Me

In 1962 Neil Simon was still a young playwright. He had scored his first Broadway hit with *Come Blow Your Horn*, and now he was adapting a play from a spoof of the "as told to" genre of celebrity biographies. *Little Me*, written by Patrick Dennis (who also wrote *Auntie Mame*), was the account of a fictional celebrity named Belle Poitrine. In Belle's quest for wealth and social status, the actress began an extravagant artistic career while being pursued by seven romantic admirers.

Neil suggested that I play all seven of Belle's suitors, there were two incarnations of one suitor, which meant eight parts. I was initially reluctant — I didn't know whether I had the energy to play all those parts. "I'm forty years old," I told him. "The timing is off." Neil was very persistent. "You're a shtarker," he told me. Neil believed in me and I believed in Neil. So I signed on.

I also got to work again with the brilliant Bob Fosse, who choreographed the play. Cy Coleman wrote the music and Carolyn Leigh wrote the lyrics. The songs in the play are still remembered today, including "Pardon Me Miss, But I've Never Done This with a Real Live Girl." The numbers included "Rich Kids Dance" and "The Other Side of the Tracks."

The show opened on November 17, 1962, at the Lunt-Fontanne Theater. It debuted during the newspaper strike, which meant no reviews and no publicity. We also competed against *Fiddler on the Roof*, *West Side Story*, and *How to Succeed in Business Without Really Trying*. We had a huge advance sale, and despite the handicaps we did very well, so much so that on November 30, 1962, *Life* magazine did a double cover with a picture of me as all of the characters. It was only the second time they'd ever done a double cover.

Little Me was a tour de force for me. I had thirty-two costume changes in the show. Some changes lasted a minute, others only a few seconds. As the Frenchman, I had a raincoat and a mustache made out of a thinly cut piece of black electrical tape. In the blink of an eye, I removed the raincoat and the mustache and was transformed into a full American colonel. I said hello and good-bye to myself three or four times in the course of the play.

The show was more than two and a half hours long and I had only a little over six minutes offstage during the entire time. That was when my costar Sven Svenson did his impressive dance number. I would lie on the little couch in my dressing room and pray for big applause, anything that would keep him on stage longer and extend my break. I would even start applauding myself and whistling to keep the applause going, so that I could have a few more moments to rest.

I was very driven and very neurotic about the play and very proud of the work I did in it. I never missed a performance, and, except for the time on stage, I generally never left my dressing room. People think that you only work two and a half hours a day doing a Broadway show. From the time I opened my eyes in the morning, I would think about how I would play the characters. You have to do that, otherwise the characters and your performance become routine and stale.

1967 Reunion Special

In 1967 Imogene, Carl, Howie, and I came together for a special on CBS. It had been thirteen years since we all worked together but it felt like we'd only been apart for a long weekend. The chemistry, the timing, and the magic were all in place.

When we walked around the studio, we could hear the whispers: "There they go." There was a tremendous amount of deference and respect toward us. We were treated like returning heroes.

As always, the show began in the

Writers' Room. Mel Brooks, Mel Tolkin, and Carl Reiner were back. Carl also brought Bill Persky and Sam Denoff, who had worked with him on *The Dick Van Dyke Show*. Again the rhythms were there. This time we could afford to take our time and polish the script. We got together two or three weeks ahead of time to write. If we didn't like a sketch, we could toss it and create another one. It was a luxury we had never known before. Still, we worked pretty quickly: We had a completed script in two weeks. *The Sid Caesar, Imogene Coca, Carl Reiner, Howie Morris Special*, as it was called, was a very balanced signature script that incorporated many of our old sketches and updated them as well. Faithful to Max's teachings, we adhered to the *Show of Shows* running order and pacing rules.

We began with a cliché sketch, which like the domestic sketches drew the audience in. Imogene plays an American tourist in Paris. She sits down next to me in an outdoor café and mistakes me for a Frenchman because I am wearing a beret. She begins to speak to me in broken French, and I answer her in fluent English.

Coca: You're a Yank!

Sid: And you're a Yankette!
Coca: Where are you from?
Sid: Gary, Indiana.
Coca: What a coincidence!
Sid: Are you from . . .
Coca: Yes, Buffalo, New York!
Sid: Isn't it a small world?
Coca: Yes, and getting smaller.
Sid: I said, Maynard, if you're going to be in Paris, you should dress like the Parasites.
Coca: And when in Rome . . .
Sid: Dress like the Romanians.

Next, Carl, Howie, and I played three sailors on a submerged nuclear submarine taking part in a test of how long people can get along. As "Operation Close Quarters" begins, the three of us couldn't be better pals. We sing together and complement each other. And we all smell nice too. After four months under water, we are ready to kill each other. Each movement by one of us gets on the other's nerves. As always, Carl's singing is a source of irritation and comedy.

We also did a fun parody of *Who's Afraid of Virginia Woolf?* called "Married Life." When we first wrote the sketch, the network was terrified of being sued. They had five lawyers rewrite it. We performed the revised sketch before an audience and didn't get one laugh. The network let us do the scene the way we had first written it.

Immy plays my wife. Her first words are, "Boy, do I hate you!" to which I respond with a heartfelt "To my true love, wherever she may be." We curse at each other and each bad word is covered by a censor's bell. When the doorbell rings, I say, "Is that the doorbell or a dirty word?"

The bell announces Carl arriving with his wife. After greeting them, asking them to sit down, and serving them drinks, I calmly ask them, "Who are you?" It turns out they are the neighbors, invited over by my wife without telling me.

I call her to come down: "Hey, Hitler! Company's here!" Immy comes down the stairs in a gold lamé suit, making her entrance with the same sultry confidence that she did in the Italian movie satires. "Do you want something to eat?" I ask the guests. "Well, you won't get it here. All she knows how to do is drink and sing off-key."

Immy responds, "Only when two people are deeply in love can they afford to hate each other like we do. That's what the maniac and I have going."

We also did a reunion of the Haircuts.

We were now spaced-out hippies, with long stringy hair and electric guitars with two and three necks. I introduce my colleagues, played by Carl and Howie: "On this side is his highness, Kabuki Goldberg. And on my remaining side is the great Lady John Edith Evans." Carl introduces me as Councilman Joseph T. Zucker and we sing our new hit, "If I Could Take a Ring and Put it on My Finger, I'd Marry Me." Where else are you going to find lyrics like, "My mother would be so happy to find out that I'm marrying a woman of the same faith as I am. Strawberry!"

We closed with the "Wastappi Opera House Presentation of Galipacci." Imogene took Nanette's role as the unfaithful wife. Once again, I played tic-tac-toe on my face. In the Earl Wild tradition of using popular melodies for the operas, we borrowed from "Makin' Whoopee," "Take Me Out to the Ballgame," the Beatles' "It's a Hard Day's Night," and closed with Petula Clark's hit "Downtown."

The show won nine Emmys, including one for writing.

Mel Redux

I worked with Mel Brooks on two movies. The first was *Silent Movie*, which was a lot of fun even though I used to be the boss and now I was part of the troupe. Mel gave me tremendous respect. When I tried scenes and business, he listened and worked with me. The chemistry between us was still there.

I also did *History of the World: Part One*. Cast as a caveman, I found a piece of business where I was hitting two stones together to make fire and I accidentally hit someone on the foot. His painful response was melodic. I discovered music. I suggested that if you got a bunch of people together and dropped rocks on their feet, you could have a chorus.

Lucy, Bob Hope, Dick Van Dyke, Milton Berle, and Danny Thomas

During my later career I had the opportunity to work with some of the legends of show business, starting with Lucille Ball. Lucy and I were social friends and we liked and respected each other very much. I got to work with her on one of her later sitcoms, and it was a wonderful experience.

You could tell right away that Lucy was the boss of that stage. She called the lighting, the camera angles, everything. Few people realize that in addition to being funny, Lucy was the head of a major studio, Desilu, which was eventually bought by Paramount. She and her husband, Desi Arnaz, were the first to film TV comedy using a three-camera system, each of which had its own film and focus. Interlocking them allowed you to shoot scenes over and over from different angles. With editing, you were able to present scenes in different ways.

Lucy was also one of the few people who really knew what comedy was. She knew what was funny and what was not and she gave me a lot of latitude on the set. If you found something, she let you go with it.

I went to Paris with Bob Hope in the late '80s to tape one of his many specials. We did one sketch together on the banks of the River Seine with Notre Dame in the background. The sketch was set in an outdoor French restaurant. I played a waiter and Bob played a patron. Every time I asked him for his order and he tried to speak, simulated bells went off (we couldn't ask the Notre Dame people to ring their bells to accommodate the shooting schedule). "You have to speak up, sir," I kept telling him. We started to yell at each other. "All I want is a cup of coffee," Bob kept saying. And the bells kept ringing.

A few days later we had an evening

performance that was taped for the special at the Paris Theater on the Champs-Elysées. When I went on I did my double-talk, starting with French. There was a buzz in the audience. They started leaning in and listening intently, which was followed by whispering. "What kind of French accent is that?" they were asking each other. When I switched to Italian, they realized what I was doing and started to laugh.

Bob was a wonderful man with a great, self-deprecating style. He remains a true American hero and will be missed.

In 1983 I worked with Dick Van Dyke on a picture called *Found Money*. It was an absolute pleasure working with that man. We played two guys who (no surprise) found a lot of money. We decided that if we saw someone doing a good deed, someone helping someone on the street, we would give them some of it. When the authorities found out, they still wanted to take us to jail.

In 1988 I worked with Milton Berle, Danny Thomas, and Morey Amsterdam in a nice little picture called *Side by Side* about newly retired friends who convince their bank to finance their dream: a shop for sportswear for senior citizens. We all worked very well together — there was no fighting and no ego. That's the way it should always be.

Drama over the Brooklyn Bridge

One of my most dramatic moments occurred in *Over the Brooklyn Bridge* (1984). It was another small film about the Jewish owner of a luncheonette on Bay Parkway in Brooklyn who dreams of owning a fancy restaurant in Manhattan. Elliott Gould played Albie, the young dreamer who needed to borrow money from his Uncle Ben (yours truly) to buy the restaurant. The only wrinkle in his plan is the family's opposition to Albie's shiksa fashion model girlfriend, played by Margaux Hemingway.

The film also starred Burt Young and Carol Kane, two wonderful actors I enjoyed working with. Carol played a cousin with a wild side everyone pushes on Elliott because she is Jewish. "A fourth cousin," I tell him, "is better than a stranger."

I got to do some good bits, variations on some of my signature pieces. When Elliott and I get into a discussion over when he is going to grow up, I tell him "when comes after later and later comes after when." When Elliott shows up at my house during a rainstorm, he hesitates to come in because

509

he's worried he'll get the furniture wet. In a variation on the old "new carpet" sketch, I pointed at the plastic slipcovers that were all over the house. "These are virgin cushions," I ad-libbed, "a battleship couldn't do damage here."

Brooklyn Bridge at its core was about unresolved anger and angst between generations. Elliott and I had a strong connection as uncle/father and son, which led to some very powerful dramatic scenes, including the denouement set at Sammy's Romanian restaurant on the Lower East Side. We ad-libbed that entire scene. I never saw Elliott Gould cry onscreen before and I don't think I ever cried before either. That's how emotional that scene was. It was a dramatic moment I never knew I had in me.

Frosch

The best job I ever had was playing Frosch the jailer in Johann Strauss's *Die Fledermaus* at New York's Metropolitan Opera House in 1987 and 1988 (the last show was on New Year's Eve, a tradition with *Die Fledermaus*). Frosch is written as a speaking part for a comedic performer, so it was a good fit for me. And they gave me a lot of latitude to inject topical humor and infuse my own style into the role. My jail-house monologue was laced with topical jokes, including references to government corruption, the Bush inauguration, and George Bush's promise not to raise taxes. "Read my lips . . ."

I still get compliments on that performance, and the reviews were very flattering. The *New York Times* wrote that "respect for tradition on Friday came from where it was least expected — from Mr. Caesar, the great American television comic who was making his house debut in this speaking part. Frosch's act III monologue operates as a kind of operatic cadenza in which action ceases and comedy is injected ad libitum. According to Viennese custom, the subject of current affairs is allowable here but only if equally applicable to Strauss's own time. Mr. Caesar alludes to the stock market, but most of his routine is admirably faithful to his surroundings and quite funny. He could give most of the opera veterans around him lessons in restraint."

The Associated Press was equally positive, calling me hilarious: "Caesar, whose forte is comic timing, used topical humor. 'It's 1887. We all remember that year. The stock market went kerplunk. I used to be chairman of Texaco. Now I'm doing this,' he said as he exited toward the cells. When a prisoner's attorney enters, Caesar greeted him. 'You're a lawyer, right? Why don't you take a shot at the Supreme Court?' And, at the point where Frosch drunkenly pretends to be two people, passing a bottle back and forth to himself, Caesar said, 'If we could find another "Little Me" we could have a nice party.' "

Imogene and After

Imogene and I worked together a number of times during our later years, and there was never a time when the magic was not there.

Many people don't know this, but Imogene became almost blind. Shadows were all she could see. But a mere detail like sight didn't impair her desire or her ability to perform. She knew my rhythm and the rhythm of the audience and that's all she needed. She was a real trouper.

When we got to a new theater, I would take her on stage and walk her from stage right to stage left and all around the stage to show her how deep it was. We would put down a huge white tape as a border to show her where the stage ended. If there was no tape, I'd have the border painted with a luminescent paint.

I will never forget how I felt when I saw Imogene on opening night. When she first walked out onto the stage, forty years just melted away. She was my partner again.

We went to different cities for eight- to ten-week engagements for almost three years with a fellow by the name of Lee Delano, who physically resembled Carl Reiner. We performed in Chicago, Boston, and San Francisco. We even played Branson, Missouri, which was like a different country. At the time, gourmet Italian food there was Chef Boyardee. We played Westwood in Los Angeles during what felt like the hottest summer in the history of the world. They wouldn't turn the air conditioning on. They claimed that the audience wouldn't be able to hear us. "Let them not hear us, but let them be comfortable while they're not hearing us," I told them to no avail. The audience stuck it out in the heat and the shows still ended with standing ovations.

Naturally we recreated some of the old sketches. We did "The Bicycle Thief" and the Hickenloopers' car crash argument. Imogene did her famous striptease. She would come out on stage wearing an overcoat and then go behind the curtain and dangle the coat very sexily with one hand where the audience could see it. She would drop the coat and she would come back out onstage wearing another overcoat, which she had had on underneath.

I recreated my in-one piece where we invited some people over to the house and the guest calls to say he's lost. I also did the expectant father sketch, in which I have a conversation with my imaginary son ("Why is the grass green? Because it isn't pink. It's green because it's green").

The Wonderful Ice Cream Suit

The Wonderful Ice Cream Suit (1998) was a picture based on a book with the same title written by the wonderful science fiction writer Ray Bradbury. Howie Morris and I were cast in small parts as owners of a men's clothing store. We were able to pick up where we left off without missing a beat, as if we had stopped working together the Friday before.

I remembered a men's clothing store at Columbus Circle down the block from International Theater, which I used to pass during the *Your Show of Shows* days. It was always going out of business — they had the sign up for years. As soon as I remembered the sign in that store, I knew how to do the scene. Howie and I came up with all of the dialogue ourselves. "Once we stop going out of business," we wailed, "we'll be out of business."

The Writers' Reunion

In 1996 the Writer's Guild sponsored a reunion of our writers, including Gary Belkin, Mel Brooks, Larry Gelbart, Sheldon Keller, Carl Reiner, Aaron Ruben, Danny Simon, Neil Simon, and Mel Tolkin. It was used as a part of a PBS pledge drive and was one of their biggest moneymakers. Getting together with the writers was a wonderful experience, and the energy of the reunion simulated what actually went on in the Writers' Room years before. The chemistry, respect, and affection were still there.

I Am Digitally Remastered

Because of breakthroughs in modern technology, I have been able to revisit my old works and digitally remaster them from old kinescopes (film versions of a live performance) so that they look better than they did when they first aired. We are introducing the old shows to generations of younger people who have only heard of us or seen clips on talk shows and retrospectives. It is interesting to revisit your work in that context. It makes you think about what you would have done differently.

I never offered my shows for syndication because I was concerned about the editing. To make nineteen-minute half hours out of one of my shows, to turn a fifty-three-minute hour into a thirty-eight-minute one, was worse than impractical, it was distasteful to me. To take the editing knife to the sketches would have killed them for me and would have deprived an audience of their full impact and comedic value.

We put our hearts and souls into the creation of those shows; we bled to create them. I wasn't about to have what we worked so hard for chopped up by editors' knives, by people who had no sense of comedy but needed to sell more commercial time. I have enough money to live on and I am more than comfortable with the level of fame I have achieved. To some people, I was part of their childhood and the golden age of television. To others I am the guy who was the coach from *Grease*. Either way, it wasn't worth compromising the completeness of the sketches.

Fortunately, in the same way that the then-new technology of television helped usher me into stardom, the digital age has allowed me to offer my work in a complete and restored format. Rather than chop the shows into pieces, I was able to distribute them as they were originally shown.

Five years ago I was approached by three talented young men, Peter Jaysen, Scott Zakarin, and Richard Tackenberg, from a company called Creative Light Entertainment. Their idea was to reissue the old shows using newly developed digital technology. I liked their creative ideas and I liked and trusted them.

Frankly, I am in awe of digitalization. The first time I went to the studio to watch the process I was struck by the level of care that went into it. It's a throwback to the old times, when everybody who worked on something wanted to be part of excellence. Good is not good enough; it has to be the best.

The first sketch I saw being digitized was "The Bavarian Clock." They split the screen for me so that I was able to compare the original version against the digitized product. On one side of the screen I saw the old version of the sketch on kinescope, with its scratches and cracks and dull visuals and patchy sound. And then on the other side of the screen I watched the new image as it was being created. The picture was clearer and cleaner than when we first did it over fifty years earlier. It was like magic. It was like having a son born again. I literally felt tears welling up in my eyes. Fifty years came back in a heartbeat. It was like I found something that I had lost and never expected to get back again. Amazing.

I've spent the last few years going through the archives, choosing and presenting sketches for public distribution. Appropriate for the digital age, I even have my own Web site, www.sidcaesar.com. While I'm certainly not pushing you to buy the old shows on video, I would not be insulted if you did. If I've learned anything over all these years, it's that a little laughter is good for the soul.

Epilogue

THE ANNIVERSARY BALL

In a recent documentary on A&E about the greatest television comedians of all time, I came in third in their ranking, after Lucille Ball and Jackie Gleason. I got phone calls from friends who were upset about third place. "I'm not running for office," I told them. I'd be happy to show in that kind of race anytime.

In the spring of 2002, NBC invited me to come to New York to be part of the network's seventy-fifth anniversary celebration. Traveling is not easy for me at this point in my life because of an inoperable hernia and other physical ailments that challenge me but do not stop me. But when I got the invitation, I felt both honored and compelled to go back to my home — the place where I grew up and came into my own. I hadn't been there in almost two years. Getting to New York was worth the effort.

Returning to New York City brought

519

back many memories. Even though I have called Beverly Hills home for over thirty years, New York is still in my blood. Everything is infused with energy and the people are alive and honest.

After a very bumpy airplane ride (which included a fellow passenger who could do double-talk in Yiddish and was not shy about showing me), Florence and I checked into our midtown hotel, which NBC had turned into a high-class dormitory for the several decades' worth of stars who came in for the event. Our thirty-fifth-floor room coincidentally or magically overlooked City Center, my old stomping grounds. Every morning for six years fifty years ago, I would grab a sandwich at the Carnegie or the Stage Deli and go to rehearsal.

Courtesy of Mel Brooks, I saw *The Producers*. I enjoyed the show, and I feel genuinely happy for Mel that he has this kind of success at this point in his life. He had left two tickets for Florence and me at the box office. I couldn't help thinking that it would have been the beginning of a great sketch if the tickets were not there. Regardless, Mel was safe. My days of hanging him out a window are long over.

Walking into the NBC studios at 30 Rockefeller Plaza on May 5, 2002, I remembered the first time I was there, back in the 1940s, to see Arturo Toscanini conducting the NBC Symphony Orchestra.

You could almost taste the frenetic New York energy and the euphoria of the event on the warm spring night, as the celebrities got out of their cars on 49th Street to cheering fans who were cordoned off in the area where the *Today Show* is now broadcast.

The red carpet was overflowing with celebrities, reporters, and camera crews. NBC's biggest stars from every decade were there — Don Adams, Bill Cosby, Robert Culp, Ted Danson, Barbara Eden, Michael J. Fox, Kelsey Grammar, Don Johnson, Jay Leno, Shelly Long, Bob Newhart, Jerry Seinfeld, William Shatner, Mr. T, Noah Wylie, and the cast of *Friends*. When a reporter asked me if I was excited, I told her that you had to be numb not to be excited about an event like this. The majesty of the evening and the event was amazing.

Jerry Seinfeld opened the show with a very funny monologue that set the tone for the evening: "Our mood is festive, our tone is self-aggrandizing . . . Almost all of the shows were ultimately canceled by the network. Ninety-eight percent of the people we are honoring here were fired. So if you think people look older than you remember them, they are actually angry."

He went on to say, "You will see the medium of television itself evolve from the little box of grainy black-and-white pictures to a big screen you could hang on the wall." He glibly added that the program was going to begin with a clip from NBC's most important decade. I respectfully disagree about the decade — they chose the 1990s.

Later in the evening, Kelsey Grammar, NBC's current biggest star, introduced me to a standing ovation. It was tough fighting back the tears. There were no statues to take home that night, but the accolades that come from my peers are all the award I need or could ever want. What talent there was in that room!

I was representing the golden age of television, as well as my colleagues and friends who are no longer with us. Among them was Pat Weaver, who had passed away a few months earlier. At two minutes to eleven, when they came back from commercial, I was standing at a podium in a tight shot. "I am going to pay tribute to those who are no longer with us in my own way." In my signature double-talk I paid tribute to Imogene Coca, Steve Allen,

Milton Berle, and Jack Benny in French, German, Italian, and Japanese.

Gene Shalit, the *Today Show* entertainment critic, told a mutual friend that seven of the ten violinists in the orchestra were young Asian women. When I lapsed into my Japanese double-talk, he watched the young women look at me quizzically, perhaps wondering why they could not quite figure out what I was saying. Fifty years later, double-talk still works its magic.

I was thinking of my successes, which were larger than writing and larger even than the comedy. They were also about the connections that were forged between families. On Saturday nights, people would have dinner together, as families. At nine o'clock, they would watch us and laugh together. For at least an hour and a half, tensions were put on hold and generations had common ground. It felt good to know that I could still reach people young and old, and make them laugh.

NBC News reported the next day that the emotional highlight of the event was the standing ovation I received. It was certainly the highlight of my evening and one of the high points of my life. The evening was a great success both for NBC and for me, with over 20 million viewers tuned in.

The next morning I started analyzing my performance and thinking about what I could have done better, and whether I could have gotten bigger laughs. I stopped before the bad habits kicked in again and just enjoyed the experience. It doesn't pay to get mad at anything anymore. That night was a *was* — and what a great *was* it was.

That afternoon I took a walk up Seventh Avenue. At 54th Street I could smell the manure wafting from Central Park, which is a pleasant smell for me because it reminds me of horses (for riding, not punching). I noticed a shoe repair shop. You don't see them in Beverly Hills. There was a time years ago when they would fix your shoes while you waited.

The Carnegie and Stage delis are still there and seem to be doing just fine. There are even more delis on that two-block strip, to capture the overflow. There is more corned beef in that two-block radius than in most of the cattle states. They used to name sandwiches after comedians and then change the names so as not to offend anyone. I don't know if there are any sandwiches that still have my name on them.

Many people came up to me in the street and thanked me not only for the night before but also for all the years of pleasure and entertainment. I in turn thanked them for watching. The trip to New York was a wonderful experience. I don't know if I'll be around for the next seventy-five years, but I'll settle for the hundredth anniversary celebration.

ACKNOWLEDGMENTS

As you know by now, I believe that both in art and in life anything done well is never done alone. I want to acknowledge the following for their help in creating this book. I would like to thank all of the talented performers I have worked with over the years, beginning with the little girl at the piano through all of my friends in the Catskills, the Coast Guard, Hollywood, Broadway, and television, including Carolyn Michel.

Florence took the brunt of my coming home hungry and worn out every night for years. She gave me dinner and calmed me down. Florence, I owe so much to you. After sixty years you still make it all possible for me. Michele Caesar helped me organize my files and pictures. I thank her for this. More importantly, I am grateful to her, Karen, and Rick for being my children.

I am also grateful to my producers and

friends at Creative Light Entertainment, Peter Jaysen, Richard Tackenberg, and Scott Zakarin, for helping to keep my legacy alive.

Drew Carey, Billy Crystal, Larry Gelbart, Richard Lewis, Carl Reiner, and Ray Romano provided kind and thoughtful words on my behalf. Thank you does not begin to cover it.

To Ron Simon at the Museum of Television and Radio for access to the archives; Jeff Abraham for his treasure trove of videotaped interviews (they brought back many wonderful memories, Jeff); Joe Franklin for his rare pictures and rarer heart; and Maria Prin who transcribed hours of taped interviews and proofread dozens of drafts and who still likes me. Thank you.

David Friedfeld, whose research assistance included hours in the subterranean archives of the New York City Public Library looking for old articles (that even the newspapers and magazines themselves no longer had). David, you're a good father, and in gratitude, now that the book is done, I am returning your son to you.

Mel Berger belies decades of jokes about William Morris agents, because he is a mensch.

Phyllis Grann, publishing industry luminary, provided invaluable input and support, which was most appreciated.

The team at PublicAffairs, consummate professionals and great people, always made me feel that both the book and I were in safe hands. Paul Golob, our first editor, got this project off the ground with enthusiasm and insight. After Paul's departure, Kenneth Turan, the *Los Angeles Times* and National Public Radio film critic, was brought in and provided essential skills and knowledge to the editing. Associate Editor (and now Editor) David Patterson, for whom this project was a Jewish baptism by fire, brought passion, wit, wisdom, and youthful energy to the book. Gene Taft was a pleasure to work with and tireless at organizing the publicity machine. I would like to offer an especially warm acknowledgment to the Publisher at PublicAffairs, Peter Osnos. Peter provided double duty on this book, not only as publisher, but also as a fan. My thanks to both of you.

And finally, Eddy Friedfeld, thank you for your absolute dedication to this book, the spirit you provided, and for all the fun we had writing it. If it's not on the page, it's not on the stage. Eddy, you did a hell of a job.